"*Mind Your Own Wellness* makes sense. It is straight-forward and easy to read. Put it to work."
—**NATUROPATHIC DR. PATRICIA BRAGG, PH.D.**
DAUGHTER OF PAUL C. BRAGG, N.D., PH.D.
(Originator of Health Food Stores) — Bragg.com

"*Mind Your Own Wellness* is simple and to the point! Highly recommended for all seeking better health."
—**DR. JOHN GRAY**
International Speaker and #1 Best-Selling Author
MEN ARE FROM MARS, WOMEN ARE FROM VENUS
MarsVenus.com

"...I strongly recommend *Mind Your Own Wellness* to all who care about their health. It is easy to read and to use as a reference book. It should be on the bookshelves of every parent. The greatest benefits of good nutrition, stress relief and exercise come from adopting what is in this book early in life, yet at any age one can benefit."
—**RUSSELL L. BLAYLOCK, M.D., C.C.N.**
Board Certified Neurosurgeon, Lecturer and Author
EXCITOTOXINS: THE TASTE THAT KILLS
BlaylockWellnessCenter.com

"*Mind Your Own Wellness* is healthy living 101. Read it from Cover to Cover!"
—**MARCI SHIMOFF**
Co-Author of the CHICKEN SOUP FOR THE SOUL series
#1 New York Times Best-Selling Author
HAPPY FOR NO REASON — MarciShimoff.com

"Most people are digging their graves with their mouths. Alex Ong teaches you the completely opposite – how to live your life with vitality, perfect health and total fulfillment."

—**PEGGY MCCOLL**
New York Times Best-Selling Author
YOUR DESTINY SWITCH
Destinies.com

"*Mind Your Own Wellness* is one of the better health/ diet/nutrition books I've read in a long time. It makes real sense, the methods are easy enough, the healthy lifestyle recommended is simple if you truly want to be "well"...and the book is as entertaining as it is easy to read!"

—**JACK ONG (no relation to author)**
Actor-Writer-Activist;
Voice Performer in such Audio books as
THE ART OF PROFITABILITY,
RICH DAD'S SUCCESS STORIES, AND
LOUIS L'AMOUR'S THE DIAMOND OF JERU
JackOng.com

"What I love about Alex's plan is that you start slow and build up to more healthy habits as you master the easy ones. That is really important in any self-help program."

—**CATHY GOODMAN, PH.D.**
Fibromyalgia Patient Activist
TheFibroConnection.com

"A healthy banquet filled with specific actions that are facts, not fads! Value-added knowledge and recommendations on every page. "

—DR. DENIS WAITLEY
International / Keynote Speaker
Best-Selling Author of THE PSYCHOLOGY OF WINNING
Co-Author of THE SECRET
Waitley.com

"*Mind Your Own Wellness* is an unique and easy to use eating strategy. Natural health shouldn't be difficult, and Alex Ong has done a wonderful job of outlining effective tips for how to eat better and get over cravings. "

—ALEXANDRA JAMIESON, CHHC, AADP
Holistic Health Counselor, Starred In SUPERSIZE ME
Author of THE GREAT AMERICAN DETOX DIET
NutritionForEmpoweredWomen.com

"This book shows you how and what to eat so you have more energy and vitality. You will learn how to lose weight, feel great, and look good!"

—BRIAN TRACY
International / Keynote Speaker
New York Times Best-Selling Author of FLIGHT PLAN
BrianTracy.com

"Insightful and knowledgeable! Alex Ong's *Mind Your Own Wellness* is a must read. It is a blueprint for any person who wants to learn the effective ways to lose weight naturally and live a healthier life."

—JOHNNY "THE TRANSITION MAN" CAMPBELL, DTM
Accredited / Keynote Speaker
Author of MOVE ON...YOUR L.I.F.E. IS WAITING
TransitionMan.com

"This book will turn the unconscious act of making poor food choices into a conscious act of making the right food choices. I love how it teaches us how to control the Inner Junkie Voice (Junk Food Voice) so it doesn't control us. Put this book in your reusable shopping bag and bring it with you to the market to help you make the right food choices."

— HOST OF THEAWARESHOW.COM LISA GARR
90.7 fm KPFK Los Angeles
98.7 fm KPFK Santa Barbara

"This book is long overdue. Anyone who regularly eats sugar and packaged, processed foods needs to read this eye-opening, hard-hitting, and ultimately inspiring book. I wholeheartedly recommend *Mind Your Own Wellness* to anyone interested in improving their health."

— BRIAN JUD
Seminar Leader, Speaker and Author
BookMarketingWorks.com

"There is a famous line in a movie *"Come with me if you want to live!"* After you read *Mind Your Own Wellness*, you will join Alex's team for better health."

— PETE CERQUA
Author of THE 90-SECOND FITNESS SOLUTION
PeteCerqua.com

"*Mind Your Own Wellness* is indeed fun to read and the steps are easy to follow. Alex Ong's 5 Color Belt Eating Formula makes creating a healthy eating regime enjoyable and effective. He's awesome!"

— KUREK ASHLEY
Peak Performance Coach and International Best-Selling Author
HOW WOULD LOVE RESPOND?
KurekAshley.com

"*Mind Your Own Wellness* is a breath of fresh air! In a very unique way, Alex Ong has created an effective and yet simple to follow eating program. Packed with tips, research and insights, this book is the perfect bridge to your path to wellness."
—**SAMANTHA GILBERT**
Certified Holistic Nutrition Practitioner
MyBodyBySam.com

"*Mind You Own Wellness* is a treasure. It is packed full of amazing insights and tips to help anyone improve or maintain excellent health. And it does not cost an arm and a leg to practice what Alex suggests. This book was a labor of love, written by a son who lost his father way too soon. It is a privilege to know Alex. He is the real deal – he really DOES want to save lives. The time you take to read this book is time invested in prolonging your life."
—**DR. DONALD C. MARTIN**
Professional Speaker, Consultant and Author
ROAD MAP FOR GRADUATE STUDY
GradSchoolRoadMap.com

"Alex Ong packs a double-wallop as a radio guest. In addition to intelligently describing his proven, commonsense 5 Color Belt Success method for improving your health, he brings authentic passion and engaging charm to this typically very serious topic. He expertly uses tongue-in-cheek humor to describe the challenges and costs of choosing to be obese, and how overeaters approach restaurant buffets with a "getting my money's worth" attitude. If you're fortunate to book Alex for your radio show, ask him to play his original composition, Greatest Hero – another example of his compassion, talent, and depth. Thank you, Alex!"
—**RADIO HOST BONNIE D. GRAHAM**
UP CLOSE & PERSONAL ON WGBB
BonnieTV.com

"This book is great for anyone who has experienced yo-yo dieting. Alex Ong explains how our thoughts could affect what and how we eat. He opens up a new door for anyone who is willing to take control of his or her Inner Junky Voice."

—DR. JOE VITALE
1# International Best-Selling Author of THE ATTRACTOR FACTOR
Co-Author of THE SECRET
MrFire.com

"Positive thinking, emotional healing and good nutrition are essential to good health. Alex has written a wonderful guide to help you get started on a journey to be the best you can be."

—BRENDA COBB
Founder and Director of The Living Foods Institute
Author of THE LIVING FOODS LIFESTYLE
LivingFoodsInstitute.com

"*Mind Your Own Wellness* identifies and de-bunks commonly accepted consumptive habits while demonstrating that many of the beliefs that we trust (or take for granted) are not harmful to our health have far reaching consequences. In a light, entertaining and fun to read format, Alex Ong offers powerful coaching solutions in an easy-to-read format with simple step-by-step instructions. A highly recommended read!"

—ELISSA MICHAUD
Publisher of THE HEALER'S GUIDE
HealerGuide.com

"*Mind Your Own Wellness* is a wonderful, down-to-earth guide to health and happiness. I found it clear and concise and perhaps most importantly, easy to implement immediately."
—**NICK ORTNER**
Executive Producer and Creator of TRY IT ON EVERYTHING
TryItOnEverything.com

"Alex Ong's Color Belt Success Formulas...much like in Martial Arts...give you the ability to start off slow and work towards becoming a wellness champion! With *Mind Your Own Wellness*, you can kick unhealthy habits' butt!"
—**BRETT BLUMENTHAL**
CEO and Founder of SheerBalance.com
Author of GET "REAL" — STOP DIETING!

"A healthy body will help you attain the confidence that, coupled with a Positive Mental Attitude, will help you achieve your loftiest goals."

– W. Clement Stone, Author, *Believe and Achieve* –
Permission granted by
The Napoleon Hill Foundation

MIND
YOUR OWN
WELLNESS

Turning Thoughts Into Reality

Alex Ong

MIND YOUR OWN WELLNESS

Alex Ong

Copyright 2008, 2010 by Alex Ong

Published by:
OCL Publishing, Inc.
Address: P.O. Box 5618, Villa Park, IL 60181

ISBN-13: 978-0-9801556-6-2
ISBN-10: 0-9801556-6-5

ISBN eBook Edition: 978-0-9801556-8-6

Library of Congress: 2007908938

Printed in the United States of America
OCL Publishing, Inc.
Villa Park, Illinois

**For educational, fund raising, business,
or special sales**

Contact: specials@MindYourOwnWellness.com

www.AlexOng.com

www.MindYourOwnWellness.com

Foreword

By

Russell L. Blaylock, M.D., C.C.N.

It was the death of my father that focused my mind on the value of good nutrition, discipline, avoiding toxins, adequate sleep and regular exercise. There are few things in life that are as traumatic as loosing a parent, especially when you are close, it is even worse when you realize that there were things that could have been done to prevent their death.

Alex Ong lost his father to a preventable disease, as did I. But, rather than ignoring the vital lessons from his tragic death, Alex sought understanding and wisdom. This book is the result of his quest. It not only turned his life around, it improved his quality of life immensely. In this most valuable book he shares what he has learned so that you too can benefit from this life-saving knowledge.

The principles in this small book are simple to follow. A great deal of knowledge concerning the causation of most diseases is pack in this volume. Nutritional science has grown enormously and we can all benefit from this new understanding of how our bodies work in response to stress, disease, poor lifestyles and bad diets.

One of the most important lessons one can learn from this book is the value of discipline. Without discipline, all is lost. We are so tempted with bad foods and drinks, lazy lifestyles and self-imposed exposure to many toxins that most just have given up and yield to the temptation. Yet, there is a heavy price to pay for this lack of will and discipline—a lifetime of illness, obesity and fatigue.

We now know that there is a strong connection between our diets and our behavior and that many of the problems we deal with concerning our children—especially as regards their bad behavior and poor learning, is based on poor diets. The lessons in this book are especially important for children from the earliest age. Changing diets by ridding them of harmful additives and inflammation producing oils and sugar can literally change a problem child into a parent's dream.

Much is now known concerning the harmful effects of food additives, many of which have been hidden by the regulatory agencies that are supposed to protect the public. Many of the additives have been shown by careful research to cause dramatic increases in cancer, degenerative brain disorders and overall poor health. Unfortunately, most physicians are not aware of many of these studies and do not warn their patients to avoid them.

Packaged, processed foods contain a large number of these additives and many enhance each other's toxicity when mixed together in a single food. My first book, Excitotoxins: The Taste That Kills, explained how the common food additive MSG and its many derivatives, can damage the developing brain of children and increase brain degeneration in adults. With neurodegenerative diseases, such as Alzheimer's and Parkinson's disease, increasing in such astronomical numbers, especially among the younger age groups, attention to these dangerous additives is critical.

Alex also points out another major problem in our society and that is our obsession with sugar. Most of us know that our children consume enormous amounts of sugar drinks and sugar-containing foods, but few are aware that the elderly are now consuming 300% more sugar than they did 20 years ago. A considerable amount of research confirms the damage done by this obsession with sugar.

While most will concede that we are eating far too many bad foods, few understand the enormous value of eating good foods, such as fruits and vegetables. In Mind Your Own Wellness, Alex shows you how to improve your intake of these life-savings and disease-preventing foods. Compelling research now confirms the enormous value of consuming a mixture of raw and cooked vegetables. Substances within these foods, called flavonoids, have been shown to powerfully inhibit cancer, prevent inflammation, dramatically reduce cardiovascular risk and protect the brain.

Stress has been shown to have a major effect on disease and poor health. We now know that chronic, unrelieved stress can cause critical areas of the brain to atrophy, leading to memory loss, clouded thinking and depression. It can also produce chronic inflammation, which is at the seat of a great many diseases of aging.

I strongly recommend this book to all who care about their health. It is easy to read and to use as a reference book. It should be on the bookshelves of every parent. The greatest benefits of good nutrition, stress relief and exercise come from adopting what is in this book early in life, yet at any age one can benefit.

-- Russell L. Blaylock, M.D., C.C.N. --
Board Certified Neurosurgeon, Lecturer and Author
"Excitotoxins: The Taste That Kills"
Advanced Nutritional Concepts, LLC
RussellBlaylockMD.com

Dedication

To lovers of health...

I hope this book helps you take control of your Inner Voices and live an awesome, healthier life.

Take your time. Eat right. And enjoy life!

All the best!

Acknowledgements
Authors, Friends, Speakers, and Families
www.AlexOng.com

It has been my luck, pleasure, and honor to come to know all of you — directly or indirectly — and I thank you for brightening my life along the way. Without your smiles or the inspiration of your books, tapes, CDs, seminars, or in-person discussions, I would not have come this far. I sincerely hope that this book could bring lights to anyone who may need it along the way. Thank You And Best Wishes To All Of You, Every Day!

- My editor Cheryl Chapman: Thank you for all your support and help, you are simply AWESOME.
- Napoleon Hill, W. Clement Stone, Don Green, and Annedia Sturgill: The Napoleon Hill Foundation – Books: *"Believe and Achieve"* and *"Think and Grow Rich"*- www.naphill.org
- Dr. T. Colin Campbell and Thomas M. Campbell - Authors: *"The China Study"*- www.thechinastudy.com
- Dr. Neal Barnard - Author: *"Food For Life"*- www.pcrm.org
- Dr. Russell L. Blaylock – Author: *"Excitotoxins: The Taste That Kills"* – www.russellblaylockmd.com
- Debby L. Anglesey - Author: *"Battling the "MSG Myth" A Survival Guide and Cookbook"*- www.msgmyth.com
- Dr. James B. Maas with Megan L. Wherry, David J. Axelrod, Barbarra R. Hogan, and Jennifer A. Blumin - Authors: *"Power Sleep"*
- Patricia Bragg, N.D., Ph.D. and Paul Bragg, N.D., Ph.D. – Authors: *"Apple Cider Vinegar"* – www.bragg.com
- Brian Tracy – Author: *"How To Raise Happy, Healthy, Self-Confident Children"* – www.briantracy.com

- Kurek and Johanna Ashley; Cori Britt; John Conger; George and Mary Foster; Dottie Georges; Charlotte Gerson; Karen Hoyos; Peter and Tamara Lowe; Andrea Metcalf; Dr. Joseph Mercola; Arnold Palmer; Theresa Puskar; Anthony Robbins; Bryan Robert; Gary Player; Kathy Smith; Sean Stephenson; Stephanie Tade; Julie Whitman; Marianne Williamson.
- Yara Abuata; Gida Aden; Bob Allen; Mike Anderson; Mike Anglesey; Rick Artus; John Assaraf; Bill Bartmann; Les and John Brown; Kelly Brownell; Katie Bushnell; Rhonda Byrne; Johnny Campbell; Jack Canfield; Alex Carroll; Jimmy Chapman; Tony Chatman; Dr. Deepak and Rob Chopra; Robert Cohen; Stephen Covey; Ethel Crisp; Harvey and Marilyn Diamond; John Dillman; Brian Dober, PGA; Maria Dorfner; Todd Duncan; Wayne Dyer; Jill Eckart; T.Harv Eker; Keith Essex; Christine Farlow; Caitilin Foley; Arielle and Debbie Ford; Karen Freschauf; Joel Fuhrman; Roger Galer; Adam Ginsberg; Ann Gittleman; Cathryn Goodman, Ph.D.; Suzanne Gratz; John Gray, Ph.D.; Deidre Hall; Mark V. Hansen; Steve Harrison; Debbie Heika; Shaun and Lori Ho; Jesse Ianniello; Alex Jamieson and Morgan Spurlock; Brian Jud; Robert and Kim Kiyosaki; John Kramer; Chiu-Nan Lai; Freddie and Emily Lam; Adrienne Lang; Dr. Brian and Lucia Larson; Bruce and Linda Lee; Debbie Lefever; Robert MacPhee; Dr. Don Martin; Peggy McColl; John McGran; Cary Miller; LuAn Mitchell; Laurie Moore; Jack Ong; Suze Orman; Dr. Dean Ornish; Nicholas and Jessica Ortner; Dr. Mehmet and Lisa Oz; Stephen Pierce; Dr. Scott Plunkett; Dan Poynter; Colin Powell; Bob Proctor; Mandi Rivieccio; Dr. Michael Roizen; Tom and Marilyn Ross; Dave Senor; Joe and Delice Serritella; Marci Shimoff; Rose Smith; Bill Sparkman; Chris Stark; Ken, Debbi, Maryssa, Kenny and Brenton Stumpf; John and MaryBeth Tedeschi; Judith VanderMerwe; Meredith Wade; Bill and Austin Walsh; Dottie and Lilly Walters; Dr. Denis Waitley; Sharon West; Leah Wilson; Oprah Winfrey; Tom Yakowicz; Glenn Yeffeth; Zig Ziglar; All my friends at Helen Plum Memorial Library.
- Linnawaty, Alicia, James, Meldon, William, and Wilton for helping me with the title of this book.

- Pat Alam; Peter and Wendy Alessandri; Dan and Joan Anderson; Walter Andrews; Charles Ann; Denis and Maila Antonio; Jimmy and Nia Antonopoulos; Lance Armstrong; Mike and Alesia Bailey; Jacque Ballard; Joon and Marilag Bautista; Robert Bell; Christie Bellino; Geoffrey Berwind; Gerald and Pat Busby; Lisa Carbonara; Ron and Robin Carlini; Jennifer Canzoneri; Pat Caputo; Jodi Carey; Tom and Maureen Carroll; Linda Carter; Anna Casas; Andy and Amy Chan; Kim Chang; Ian Cheney; Bee Cheng; Grace Cheng; Fong C. Choon; Kan Chou; Dave Cogozzo; Carol Cooling; David Corbin; Kim Cordy; Tom and Michelle Cummins; Judy Curtis; Betty Cyr; Rich Darnell; Paul and Nicci Davis; Bill and Judy Degnan; Richard and Angelica DelValle; Anna Diaz; Mary Donovan; Julie Edgin; Rickie and Anne Ellis; Wendy Ellis; Gilbert and Analiza Enriquez; Caldwell Esselstyn; Audrey Eufrasio; Jim Fergle; Chris and Wendy Ferguson; Jim and Kathleen Fleming; Ashley Ganski; Joe Garrett; Peter Gault; Teno and Diana Geritano; Frances Gilles; Julie Gillman; Matt and Kirsten Gillono; Tony Goben; Seth Godin; Hesh Goldstein; Sensei Bob and Judy Griffith; Bo Grin; Jeff and Christy Gruskovak; Amy Hall; Bonnie Hamlin; Darren Hardy; Kevin and Susan Hay; Dean and Laura Holmes; Robyn Hessinger; Sung and Solana Hong; Tony Hsieh; Bonnie Hunt; Mary Hurley; Jia and Pin Hwang; Oh Hwee; Elaine Jackson; Karen Johnson; Rodney and Michelle Johnson; Pam and Tracey Jones; Larry King; Garrett and Steve Kroschel; Mike Koenigs; Joyce Kosasih; Claudia Krauspe; Larry and Vivian LaBorn; Jacki Lawyer; Horace and Tracy Lai; Wayne Lemon; Jason Liller; Sally MacLean; Dave Malave; Gary Mallek; Judith Mathewson; Barb Mazzochi; Marc McCutcheon; Nancy Means; Paul and Barb Mehlhaff; Rebecca Miarnowski; Kenny Mitchell; George Mui; Henky Mulyono; Sammy Murugaya; Mike and Deb Nangle; Beth O'Conner; Edward and Vivian Ooi; Tom and Lynn Ostdiek; Mustapha and Rosalinda Ouchen; Linda Palek; Gary and Kyoko Pang; Tom and Jeanine Parrillo; Ken and Holly Patete; Tom Pearcy; Betty Perry; Danielle Pierre; Glenn and Rebecca Placek;

Chuck and QiuMei Pollock; Frank and Yunling Prang; Teresa Pudi; Donna Puscheck; Carlito and Amelita Quiatchon; Chip Rank; Dr. John Robbins; Pete Reyes; Myra Robinson; Mark and Sue Roucka; Effendy Salim; Dr. Kumar and Savita Sahbarwal; Bob Salter; Penny Sansevieri; Carrie Savickas; Linda Schehl; Eric Schlosser; Don, Dick, and Greg Schroeder; Kevin and Kathy Schuele; Tom and Cathy Schweighardt; Chow Y. Seng; Vikas Sheth; Sandra Simon-Nichols; Deanna Sipe; Zifa Smajic; Jeffrey Smith; Suzanne Somers; Robert and Janis Stob; Sally Strange; Gary and Nancy Stratton; Marlene Stratton; Laura Subianto; Kristin Sunderhalf; Paula Tammen; Larry and Sally Tantilla; Cheryl Tiede; Shirly Tirta; Pablo Tobiano and Maureen Sadsad; Ed and Kim Topol; Cherylee Trenkamp; Trung Truong; Mike Udoni; Al and Susie Utacht; Jesse and Marcy Vargas; Maria Vazquez; Sarah Victory; Greg Vogt; Cindy Ward; Dr. Stacia Wert-Gray; William and Pam White; Judith Williamson; Eric and Lynda Wilson; Bob and Marianne Wolfe; Christina, Olive, and Victor Wong; Tim and Winni Yang; Wang Yun; Khalid and Iffat Zafar; Megan Zehnder and many Relatives and Friends not mentioned, thanks a million!

- Lao Pa Lin Zhong Guo; Koh Jee; Mommy Frances Barrows and Mommy Twyla Winterhalter (Who took care of my wife and I during our college years while we were far away from our parents); Alvin Ong; James, Alicia (My dearest sister Ong Lay Ching), Meldon, and Melody Wee; Godparents Renty Susanto and Nuraida Tjiam; Cita and Indah Megasuri; Mom Moi Hwa and Mom-In-Law Soei Young (Who gave myself and my wife their unconditional love and care); our two very Sweet and Understanding Sons William and Wilton; and last but not least, my lovely wife Linnawaty (Who turned me from a study challenged student into someone who loves to study, read, and write).

In Memory Of My Dearest Daddy and Golfing Buddy
Ong Choon Lee!
"Without you, I would have none of the above."
"Daddy! You Are My Greatest Hero!"
Alex Ong - OCL Publishing, Inc.

Disclaimer

The author has made every attempt to make this book as precise and complete as possible; however, there may be misprints or typographical errors. The information provided in this book contains the opinions, research, personal experience, and thoughts of its author. The author is not a medical doctor. None of the information should be used as a substitute for the advice of a qualified health professional. Do not use any of the suggestions or recommendations in this book without first consulting with your doctors, especially if you are undergoing medical treatments or have had medical treatments in the past. You should consult a certified health professional and be monitored throughout the process. Results may vary. Taking on any of the suggestions or recommendations from this book must be done at your own risk. The author, editors, agents, publishers, or employees, expressly disclaim all responsibility for any adverse effects, liability, loss, or damage of any form, directly or indirectly due to the use of any information in this book.

How To Contact The Author

- Keynote / Speaking engagements
- Individual or group coaching
- Tele-seminars

"When stress, weight, or healthcare cost happens to soar, Alex Ong is the guy to call!" To discuss hiring the author for your next special event, conference, or fund-raiser, contact:

Alex Ong
Keynote Speaker
Natural Health Author
630-673-6268

OCL Publishing, Inc.
P.O. Box 5618, Villa Park, IL 60181
Alex@MindYourOwnWellness.com

Contents

Introduction:

"Most of us are fortunate to be born healthy. It is what we have learned and have chosen to put into our mouths that drove our bodies crazy."

The goal of this book is to help you better understand that what you are just about to put into your mouth will affect how you feel and look. Like it or not, that is the way it is.

How can MIND YOUR OWN WELLNESS help?

Chapter 1 is a wake up call for all of us (adults and children) in America!

Chapter 2 will show you the "GOODs or BADs" of 14 Common Things that you and your family eat and drink — including *Milk, Sugar-Free products, Fat-Free Foods, and more...*

Chapter 3 explains the benefits of organic foods.

Chapter 4 will provide you with more than 30 essential tips to help you along the way.

Chapter 5's title says it all: It's time to face the fact! What Is Your Current BMI?

Chapters 6 to 9 will show you how to turn your thoughts into reality by getting to know your Inner Twin Voices; your Inner Healthy Voice and your Inner Junky Voice. You will learn how to take control over your Inner Junky Voice and how to handle external forces, such as mouth-watering junk-food advertisements, peer pressure, etc.

Chapter 10 will provide you with three approaches to "Say NO" to your Inner Junky Voice.

Chapter 11 shows you how "Advertisements" and your Inner Junky Voice go against you.

Chapters 12 and 13 will enhance your understanding about wellness! Besides eating right and exercising regularly, proper breathing and resting (sleeping) are also crucial to help you improve your health.

Chapter 14 will remind you how One Action could change your life!

Chapters 15 and 16 will show you how to put your thoughts into action. In addition, the 5 Color Belts' Success Formulas will guide you to eat and fill your stomach with healthy foods first and leave a little or no room for junk food – *No starving, guaranteed!* Once you learn the ways to control your thoughts and start taking action, you too will begin to lose pain and extra weight — a pound at a time. You will also replace bad eating habits with good ones, such as,

- Not overeating
- Leaving junk food for entertainment or treat purpose and eating more healthy foods

Most importantly, at the end of the day, you will learn to love your new body and your new image. You will not want to go back to your old habits because you will be in charge of your body and your thoughts.

Soon, you will realize that it is really not that easy to become overweight or obese and to stay that way. You will have to be totally committed and truly determined consciously or subconsciously to stay overweight by spending hundreds of dollars on unhealthy food, diet pills, or Liposuction surgeries, and stressing yourself physically and mentally. How about saving your hard earned dollars for your retirement, instead?

Can you imagine how much you could save per month, per year, or in 10 years, if you cut down your junk food expenses by 80%? Most importantly, what would happen to your priceless body, health, and emotions?

This book is *short and easy to read.* Bring it and use it as a reminder while doing your grocery shopping. Have fun doing it!

"To jump start with the 5 Color Belts' Success/Eating Formulas, go to www.MindYourOwnWellness.com/quickstartguide.html right now and download your free Quick Start Guide."

1
How Is Our Health, America?

The following data was obtained from one of the giants in the field of nutrition science, Dr. T. Colin Campbell, from the book he coauthored, "The China Study."[1]

The nearly 300 million people in our country are not well. The shocking statistics for American adults are as follows:

- 82% have at least one risk factor for heart disease
- 81% take at least one medication during any given week
- 50% take at least one prescription drug during any given week
- 65% are overweight
- About 105 million (one in every three) have a dangerously high cholesterol level of 7 (defined as 200mg/dL or higher)
- About 50 million have high blood pressure
- Over 63 million have pain in the lower back (in large part related to circulation and excess body weight, both influenced by diet and aggravated by physical inactivity) during any given three-month period
- Over 33 million have a migraine or severe headache during any given three-month period
- 23 million had heart disease in 2001
- At least 16 million have diabetes
- Over 700,000 died from heart disease in 2000
- Over 550,000 died from cancer in 2000
- Over 280,000 died from cerebro-vascular diseases (stroke), diabetes, and Alzheimer's in 2000"

What About Youths In America?

- Roughly one in three youths in America (ages six to nineteen) is already overweight or at risk of becoming overweight

How could this have happened to America? We are suffering from the so-called "disease of abundance." We have access to a huge variety of foods, both healthy and unhealthy; and we tend to eat more than we need. In addition, many of us have the habit of sitting and watching numerous hours of TV programs every day and we don't move very much.

"According to the A.C. Nielsen Co., the average American watches more than four hours of TV each day (or two months of nonstop TV-watching per year) ...According to an American Journal of Public Health study, an adult who watches three hours of TV a day is far more likely to be obese than an adult who watches less than one hour."[2]

Consciously or subconsciously, we also allowed ourselves to be freely influenced by advertisements that affect our decisions, such as, what and how we should eat, what we should wear, what car to drive, and more.

Generations ago, when meat, regular sugar, and other toxic food ingredients were scarce or non-existent, diseases such as cancer, heart attack, and diabetes were not common. In today's society, cancer, heart attack, diabetes, and other diseases have become one of the main topics of the day. We may hear, "so and so just made it through his or her heart bypass," "so and so did not make it," "so and so just had a kidney removed," "so and so is now going through chemotherapy," "so and so has to take medicine for life and the medicine is giving him or her so much pain," or "so and so only has X number of years, months, weeks or days to live."

As Dr. T. Colin Campbell and Mr. Thomas M. Campbell stated in their book *The China Study,*

> *"Animal protein, even more than saturated fat and dietary cholesterol, raises blood cholesterol levels in experimental animals, individual humans, and entire populations. International comparisons between countries show that populations subsisting on traditional plant-based diets have far less heart disease, and studies of individuals within single populations show that those who eat more whole, plant-based foods not only have lower cholesterol levels, but, have less heart disease.*
>
> *Never before have we had such a depth of understanding of how diet affects cancer both on the cellular level as well as a population level. Published data show that animal protein promotes the growth of tumors. Animal protein increases the levels of a hormone, IGF-1, which is a risk factor for cancer, and high-casein (the main protein of cow's milk) diets allow more carcinogens into cells, which allow more dangerous carcinogen products to bind to DNA, which allow more mutagenic reactions that give rise to cancer cells, which allow more rapid growth of tumors once they are initially formed. Data show that a diet based on animal-based foods increases a female's production of reproductive hormones over her lifetime, which may lead to breast cancer."*[3]

Clue: Shift your regular diet towards more plant-based foods and cut down on animal protein, including dairy products and lean meat, to at least minimize the chance of getting cancer or to slow down the speed of cancer growth.

How can MIND YOUR OWN WELLNESS come into play? Once you learn to draw upon your Power of Thought to guide your Inner Twin Voices (Inner Healthy Voice and Inner Junky Voice) in Chapter 7, you will increase your odds to control your thoughts and start taking actions; which could put you back on track to start losing pain and extra pounds.

Take control of your Thoughts (your Inner Healthy and Junky Voices), and keep your External Influences away from you and you will start to feel and look great. Take Action, Take Control – Put Less Unhealthy Food Into Your Mouth. How? Let's Get Started!

2
Getting Started

Know a little more and live better...

Read Your Food Ingredients Whether You Like It Or Not – Start with the so-called "OK-TO-EAT" foods in your kitchen, pantries, and refrigerator.

"Know The 14 Common Things To Minimize! Cut It Down If It Makes Sense To You!"

1) My Milk or Your Milk?

Is milk good for you? It doesn't matter what kind of cow's milk it is, drink a little less and you may feel better. Just like everything else, use milk and dairy products in moderation.

Common short-term side effects of milk and dairy products are:

- Respiratory problems or Asthma
- Sinus (running nose or excess mucus in the throat)
- Skin rashes
- Diarrhea
- Vomiting
- Ear infections
- Bronchitis or sore throat
- Body aches and pains

Potential long-term side effects:

- Increase in cholesterol — leading to heart problems
- Increase in saturated fat
- Kidney problems from dairy foods that are high in fat and salt
- Increase the chance of getting cancer

Fun MILK Quiz: Ask a friend!

1. *How do you pronounce M-I-L-K?*
2. *Ask your friend to pronounce MILK as fast as they can, for 10 times.*
3. *Once the 10ᵗʰ MILK is pronounced, ask your friend, "What do cows drink?"*

You are likely to hear the answer, "MILK" most of the time.

Correct Answer Is: Water

First of all, we need to recognize that milk and dairy products may not be as good as we thought. As stated in Dr. Neal Barnard's book, *Food for Life*:

> *"Dairy products are not the solution to osteoporosis... Milk is largely ineffective in slowing bone loss. The high occurrence of osteoporosis has more to do with the excess of protein Americans eat, along with a sedentary life-style and tobacco and alcohol use, than with any 'deficiency' of cow's milk."*[4]

Instead of helping you get stronger, many dairy products (excluding skim milk, certain yogurt and other nonfat dairy products) could actually add a portion of cholesterol and saturated fat into your body. Not to mention the delicious, yummy cheese that is also loaded with salt, which could bring even more harm to your body if it is overeaten. For example, a ham, cheese, and egg sandwich with a couple of glasses of milk for breakfast; a double cheese burger with fries and soda for lunch; and deep-fried chicken, fish, or shrimp, fries, and a cup of milk shake for dinner would be overdoing it.

If you or your children are currently suffering from asthma or other respiratory problems, it could be because of milk allergies. Unfortunately, many people who are sensitive to dairy products are unaware of the causes to their problems.

So, how much milk do you need to drink to get enough calcium for your body? Just minimize it whenever you can because milk is actually best for calves (baby cows, not humans!). Drinking a few glasses of milk per week (as treats) is more than enough. How about three glasses of milk per day? That is on the very high side.

"By eating calcium-rich vegetarian foods, including leafy green vegetables such as broccoli and kale, white beans, and juices, and a variety of fruits and vegetables, you can obtain all the calcium your body needs. But keeping your bones strong and avoiding osteoporosis depends more than calcium intake — you also need to keep calcium in your bones...while animal protein, excess salt and caffeine, and tobacco can cause calcium loss."[5]

Lesson 101 from Moo...Moo... (we could actually learn from cows) is:

"Drink more water and eat more plant-based foods in order to get the natural calcium."

Natural calcium substitutes can be found in the following:[6]

Vegetables	Calcium (mg)
Broccoli (1 cup, boiled)	178
Collards (1 cup, boiled)	148
Kale (1 cup, boiled)	94
Squash, butternut (1 cup, boiled)	84
Sweet potatoes (1 cup, boiled)	70
Onions (1 cup, boiled)	58
Brussels sprouts (8 sprouts)	56
Celery (1 cup, boiled)	54
Carrots (2 medium)	38
Cauliflower (1 cup, boiled)	34
Potato, baked (1 medium)	20
Romaine lettuce (1 cup, boiled)	20

Legumes	Calcium (mg)
White beans (1 cup, boiled)	161
Pinto beans (1 cup, boiled)	82

Green beans (1 cup, boiled)	58
Lima beans (1 cup, boiled)	52
Kidney beans (1 cup, boiled)	50
Lentils (1 cup, boiled)	37

Grains	**Calcium(mg)**
Wheat Flour (1 cup)	49
Wheat bread (1 slice)	30
Brown rice (cooked, 1 cup)	23

Fruits	**Calcium (mg)**
Figs, dried (10 medium)	269
Navel Orange (1 medium)	56
Raisins (2/3 cup)	53
Pear (1 medium)	19
Apple (1 medium)	10
Banana (1 medium)	7

2) High "Animal Protein" Anyone?

Do your current breakfasts, lunches, and dinners consist of mainly animal protein, such as the following?

- Milk
- Eggs
- Bacon
- Cheese
- Sausages
- Burgers
- Steaks
- Fried chicken or meat

Animal protein is often high in saturated fat and cholesterol. The following are the reasons why high animal protein diets are not the best for our bodies:

1) *High-protein foods cause calcium to be lost in the urine.*[7]
2) *High-protein foods also release by-products that act as diuretics, forcing the kidneys to work much harder than they should, gradually wearing out the nephrons, which are the kidney's filter units.*[8]
3) *Excess protein in the diet actually interferes with the absorption and retention of calcium and prompts the body to excrete calcium, laying the ground for brittle bones. This excretion occurs because animal proteins, including milk, make the blood acidic. The body pulls calcium from the bones to balance that condition.*[9]

However, *"not all proteins had the same effect. What protein consistently and strongly promoted cancer? Casein, which makes up 87% of cow's protein, promoted all stages of cancer process."* And *"people who eat the most animal-based foods got the most chronic disease."*[10]

It is true that protein is important to the body; but if your main protein source only comes from meat and dairy products instead of plant-based protein, it could speed up your chance of getting some forms of cardiovascular disease, such as high blood pressure, stroke, and/or heart disease. Therefore, it is important for us to eat more plant-based protein and reduce the intake of animal protein to the minimum.

In case you are suffering from some form of cardiovascular disease, *"The most dramatic recent finding is that heart disease can be prevented and even reversed by a healthy diet."*[11] Therefore, if you were to convert your animal-based food to plant-based food, you would likely see a positive change to your health. However, the choice is absolutely yours. No one can change your eating habits unless you choose to do so.

3) Saturated Fat:

If you love to eat animal fat because that is what makes meat extremely juicy and tender, or oily deep-fried foods, you have taken the first step towards the Heart Attack Club, because saturated fat is known to increase bad cholesterol (LDL). Research has shown that even the leanest beef, pork, or chicken breast is already full of saturated fat. However, eating lean meat is certainly better than eating fatty meat. Just remember the key word: Moderation.

Saturated Fat is commonly found in:

- Chicken (Including lean meat)
- Pork (Including lean meat)
- Beef (Including lean meat)
- Lamb (Including lean meat)
- Chocolate
- Cookies
- Sweet and salty snacks
- Frozen and prepared foods
- Ice cream
- Cheesecakes
- Desserts
- Butter
- Cheese and other dairy products
- Burgers
- Fried foods
- Lard (animal fat)
- Salad dressings
- Vegetable cooking oil

Common side effects:

- Weight gain
- Loss of energy
- Stiff neck

- Body aches and pains
- Increase in bad cholesterol (LDL)
- Strokes
- Heart attack
- Other health diseases

"Our bodies make plenty of cholesterol for our needs and we do not have to add any."[12] In case you enjoy cooking with palm oil, palm kernel oil, coconut oil, or eating food made with them, think again! They are among the top three winners in high saturated fat count.

Even though all other kinds of so-called healthier vegetable oils (by far the best – olive oil) are lower in saturated fat than lard (animal fat), palm oil, palm kernel oil, and coconut oil, it is not recommended to overuse any of them. Minimize your use whenever you can.

4) Trans Fat:

Do partially hydrogenated vegetable oil and fully hydrogenated vegetable oil sound familiar? These are the kinds of vegetable oil that are chemically saturated by a process called hydrogenation. Adding hydrogen into vegetable oil to solidify it creates this form of oil.

Other common names:
- Partially hydrogenated cottonseed oil
- Partially hydrogenated soybean oil
- Partially hydrogenated coconut oil
- Fully or partially hydrogenated vegetable oil

Trans fat is usually found in:
- Deep fried foods (fries, chicken, cheese balls, chips, pie crust, and fruit pies)
- Peanut butter (some low fat ones too)
- Margarine
- Vegetable shortenings
- Chocolate
- Cookies
- Crackers
- Cakes
- Candies
- Cream
- Potato or vegetable chips
- Fruits or vegetable pies
- Frozen foods

Many food manufacturers use hydrogenated oils because it increases the shelf-life of the products in the grocery store. However, if you were to eat food made out of trans fat on a regular basis, it will not help *you* live longer.

How harmful is it to your body?

Trans fats are one of the major causes of heart attack, strokes, and other heart problems. If you would love to live a healthier life, avoid it or at least, minimize it. It is known for lowering your good cholesterol (HDL) and increasing your bad cholesterol (LDL) and your overall cholesterol level. Soon, it will put you on the highway to heart trouble by clogging your arteries. If the artery going to your brain is blocked, you will have a stroke and if the artery going to your heart is clogged, you will have a heart attack. Take your choice; which artery do you prefer to have blocked? It's not much of a choice, so avoid these foods as much as possible.

Look At The Very Fine Print:

If there is a label on the food package that says, **"No Trans Fat,"** look a little closer to see if there is a very fine print that reads, **"*per serving."** A serving usually equals to 1 to 2 tablespoons or 7 to greater than 32 grams. When **"*per serving"** is stated, it is a clue to you that by eating 3 to 4 servings, you would have eaten some Trans Fat. If you finish eating the whole package or container of **"No Trans Fat – Per Serving,"** you would have actually added quite a bit of trans fat into your body. After years of consistent and persistent efforts of "having to" eat that unhealthy food with **"No Trans Fat – Per Serving,"** you may have earned yourself a Free Lifetime Membership to the "Heart Attack Club" without knowing it. For this reason, various restaurants and food companies have already stopped, or at least limited, the use of ingredients that contain Trans Fat.

5) MSG (Monosodium Glutamate)

MSG could also show up in foods under the following common names:

- Accent
- Autolyzed yeast
- Amino acid
- Autolyzed plant protein
- Calcium caseinate
- E621
- Flavor enchancer
- Gourmet powder
- Gutamic acid
- Hydrolyzed vegetable protein
- Monopotassium glutamate
- Sodium caseinate
- Vetsin
- Yeast Extract

What is it?

MSG or Monosodium Glutamate, is a type of food additive commonly known as flavor enhancer. Its look and size is very much like sugar and salt, except that it is long in shape rather than crystallized cubes like sugar and salt. But, when dissolved in water, it is invisible! Its job is to deceive your taste buds by making the food taste better than it is. It also makes you eat more than you need. Sound familiar? What will happen when you eat more than you need all the time? You will become overweight, obese, and threatened by heart disease!

How does it affect you?

"MSG excites not only the taste buds, it also excites nerve cells, eventually damaging and killing them... The distribution of

cellular damage caused by large concentrations of MSG is very similar to that seen in human cases of Alzheimer's disease."[13] In other words, through long-term use, it could be harmful to the brain and nervous system.

The following are some of the **common side effects of MSG** based on Debby Anglesey's *Battling the "MSG Myth" – A Survival Guide and Cookbook,*[14] Dr. Blaylock's *Excitotoxins: The Taste That Kills* books, and my personal experience:

- Abdominal discomfort
- Angina (pain in and around heart and ribs)
- Anxiety or panic attacks
- Arrhythmias (which could lead to stroke)
- Asthma symptoms
- Bloating
- Chest pain
- Chronic cough
- Constipation
- Dehydration
- Dizziness
- Fatigue
- Extreme thirst
- Heart palpitations (irregular heart beat)
- Hair loss
- Hyperactivity – especially in children
- Loss of concentration and energy
- Migraine headache
- Mood swing
- Runny nose
- Shortness of breath
- Sore throat
- Sudden energy loss
- Tingling or numbness on face, ears, arms, legs or feet
- Urge to eat until stomach hurts
- Vomiting

MSG is commonly found in:

- Canned soups and foods
- Sausages
- Most flavored potato chips and other salty snack foods (Including children's snacks)
- Chips' dips
- Packaged chicken and beef stocks
- Frozen and processed foods
- Instant noodles' seasonings

How to reduce my intake of MSG?

If you are currently a heavy user of the above MSG products, the following could help:

1) Choose 100% organic products or at least 100% natural products.
2) Switching your current eating habits using the 5 Color Belts' Success Formulas in Chapter 16 could reduce your MSG consumptions naturally. How much MSG do you wish to cut out off your meals? The choice is yours! You could cut 10% by using the White Belt's Success Formula or you could cut 80% or more by using the Red or Black Belt's Success Formula.

Plus, read those labels carefully. Minimize the purchase of products that contain MSG or its hidden names. If you are in the habit of eating out, you probably have consumed a portion of MSG because numerous restaurants, including fast food restaurants use MSG to make food taste better. It's best to ask to be sure! On the other hand, other restaurants are busy promoting their "NO MSG" menus to attract customers who are sensitive to MSG. So, whenever possible, do not add more MSG into your body with your restaurant food or take-home snacks.

How do you know if your favorite restaurants are using MSG?

1. Ask the restaurant owner or manager if they use MSG.
2. Cross-reference with the *MSG's Common Side Effects* listed above. Take note of how you feel during and after your eat-out meal. The side effects could start as soon as 15 minutes and last for more than 24 hours.

6) Table Sugar or Regular Sugar

Sugar in other common forms or names:

- Dextrose
- Fructose
- Glucose
- High fructose corn syrup
- Saccharose
- Sucrose
- Sweetener
- Syrup

Is sugar really fat free?

Before you eat it, yes sugar is fat free! But once you eat it, it will turn into fat if you don't burn it off shortly after your consumption. As stated in the book, *You On A Diet* by Michael F. Roizen, M.D. and Mehmet C. Oz, M.D.:

> *"Simple sugars (as in cola): When sugar, which is quickly absorbed and sent to the liver, meets the liver in the digestion process, the liver tells your body to turn that sugar into fat if it can't be used immediately for energy."*[15]

So, is sugar really fat free? Now you know, it is not!

Potential or common side effects:

- Anxiety
- Aging
- Bloating
- Hyperactivity in children
- Constipation
- Heart diseases
- Fatigue

- Diabetes
- Obesity
- Food craving
- Lack of focus or concentration (leads to decrease productivity)
- Tooth decay
- Lost concentration
- Lack of ability to sit still
- Premature aging and wrinkles
- Weight increase leading to health challenges
- Weakened immune system — get sick more easily and frequently
- Difficulty sleeping — especially for children

In case you are not aware, high concentrations of sugar can also be found in the following:

- Canned foods
- Adults and children's canned and boxed fruit juice, soda, and cereal
- All kinds of sweet snacks, pastries, and baked goods
- Fat free yogurt and ice cream
- Energy bars
- Energy drinks

How To Minimize?

Purified, distilled, or filtered water is by far the best thirst quencher. By drinking water, you could cut down your sugar intake by 35 grams (approximately 1 can of sugar soda) to 140 grams (approximately 4 cans of sugar soda) or more per day. Depending on how many cans of sugary soda you drink each day, you will also eliminate those unwanted colorings, preservatives, toxic materials, and excess salts from your body.

Therefore, start today by gradually working pure drinking water into your healthy habits and phasing out sugar drinks whenever you can. The sooner you reduce your sugar consumption, the faster your body will help you stay healthy by strengthening your immune system and lowering your weight.

If you can cut your sugar intake by 35 grams (1 can of sugar soda) per day, it will add up to cutting down your sugar intake by approximately *28 pounds per year*.

Let's do the math:

35 grams of sugar per 12oz soda x 365 days = 12, 775 grams of sugar

Take 12,775 grams divided by 454 grams (a pound) = ***28.13 pounds of sugar per year!***

Can you imagine how much better you will feel from simply cutting out one can of soda per day?

By the way, our bodies do not need that extra supply of table sugar to function properly. As long as you are eating enough fresh fruits and vegetables, you are getting all the sugar your body needs.

Advantages of eating more fresh fruits and vegetables:

- Give your body the natural fiber to help with digestion and elimination
- Boost your immune system to keep you away from sickness
- Improve your concentration
- Improve your mood

- Achieve anti-aging benefits
- Overall better health ...Priceless!

Minimize your table or regular sugar intake whenever possible. Choose organic sugar over refined sugar for the following reasons:

- Human nature: Organic sugar is 2 to 3 times more expensive than regular sugar. The more expensive it gets, the less you are likely to use it. Consciously or subconsciously, you will feed yourself and your family or friends less sugar.
- Health reasons: Organic sugar contains no artificial additives or preservatives, which are harmful to your body.

7) Salt

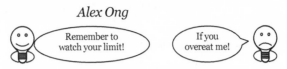

Salt is one of our bodies' requirements. However, it should only be taken in moderation, that is, between 1.2 grams to less than or equal to 5.8 grams of salt for an adult — depending on your current health condition. If you overdose on it consistently, it will automatically enroll you into the "High Blood Pressure Club."

> *"It is estimated that about 50,000,000 adults in America has high blood pressure (hypertension)."*[16]

According to the popular website: *www.wikipedia.org*, the following are recommended salt intake levels from three countries in grams per day for an adult:

New Zealand:

Adequate Intake 0.46g to 0.92g sodium = **1.2g to 2.3g salt** per day

- Upper Limit 2.3g sodium = **5.8 g salt** per day

Australia:

The recommended dietary intake is 0.92g to 2.3g sodium per day (= **2.3g to 5.8g salt**)

United States:

The 2005 *Dietary Guidelines for Americans* suggested that adults in the US should consume **less than 2.3g of sodium** (or **less than 5.8 g salt**) per day.

Common side effects for eating too much salt:

- Weight increase because excess salt retains water in your body
- Kidney problems
- Hypertension (High blood pressure)

Is hypertension or high blood pressure dangerous? Certainly! Hypertension could lead to the following:

- Strokes
- Heart problems or other heart diseases

Salts' camping grounds:

- Canned meat (Fish, Chicken, Beef, Pork), vegetables, or sauces
- Frozen processed foods
- Preserved foods
- Salty snacks
- Soda
- Canned vegetable drinks
- Sausages
- Cheeses

Once again, plant-based food (not from canned) is still the best bet for better health.

How Salt and Sugar Work Together

Your body is always looking for balance. For example, after you have consumed a good portion of salty snacks, your body (Inner Junky Voice – Chapter 7) will demand you to drink a big cup of sugary soda or vice versa.

Popular Real Life Example: What do you usually eat at a movie theatre? The more popcorn you wolf down, the thirstier you will be. So, the more sugary soda you will drink and then the more sweet treats you will eat. How do you usually feel after you are done with the movie and consuming all that junk? GUILTY! Best bet: minimize *both* salt and sugar consumption altogether! If you really have to eat that popcorn and drink that soda while watching your favorite movies, buy the smallest size (forget about paying a few cents more to double the size); you know by now that free junk food refills are not a good option either.

8) Caffeine

Dear Parents or Future Parents,

Do you know that you may have accidentally loaded up your children with caffeine every day and then wondered why they were so out of control at home or at school?

Caffeine is one of the "Three Musketeers: — Caffeine, Sugar, and MSG" that could be the major cause of your child's hyperactive behavior both in school and at home. If you allow your child to drink soda (sugar and caffeine), eat chocolate (sugar and caffeine), and flavored sweet or salty snacks (MSG) every day, the "Three Musketeers" could be the clue to your child's wild behavior.

By educating and showing your child the benefits of replacing soda with water, chocolate with fresh fruit snacks and treats without MSG, you will be pleasantly surprised with the results over time. Children are born sweet and loving. It is often what we feed them, and what we allow them to watch and learn, that mold their behaviors. Be patient! In order to show your child the right way to eat, you must first lead by example.

How would caffeine affect an adult?

Common side effects of caffeine plus cream and sugar (from coffee, chocolate, energy pills or drinks, soda):

- Mood swing
- Dehydration
- Nervousness
- Quick/ hot temper
- Impatient

Combining caffeine and sugar together (this commonly happens with soda, energy pills, or drinks like sweetened coffee) could be the reason you often get a sudden surge of energy that causes you to lose concentration and makes you need to move around instead of sitting still long enough to get a short project done in one sitting. In addition, once the doubled-up energy is over, you will experience the doubled-down impact — just like a roller coaster.

To make the scene even cuter, once your energy runs out, you are likely to go for a second or third round of caffeine and sugar to keep yourself "up" until day's end. You could call this form of ups and downs "The Stock Market."

For some people, drinking a cup of coffee (8oz) a day makes them feel great for the rest of the day and that is fine; however, if you have to depend on two, three, four, or five cups of coffee per day, then you are off the moderation chart. Once again, the choice is yours.

Suggestion: Sleep eight hours or more per night and you might not need caffeine and sugar as much to wake you up during the day. If you really like coffee, why not let it be your "morning treat" rather than your "Wake Up, Stay Up" drug which will also ruin your sleep at night?

9) Nitrite

If you are a big fan of canned meat, bacon, ham, sausages, and hot dogs, and you eat them regularly, you might want to re-think this practice. Yes, they certainly taste good and are easy to prepare. Just open, heat, add buns with toppings, eat a few, and voila! Your meal is done!

There is a common saying that "Time Is Money!" No doubt about it, but saving time without eating right could cost you more money in the long run.

Not only are canned meat, bacon, ham, sausages, and hot dogs high in salt, which you already know is not the best for your health, a large percentage of them also contain Nitrite, a preservative which is known to cause cancer in experiments with rats. Even though human studies have not been performed, *"it is likely that a chemical such as this, which consistently causes cancer in both mice and rats, can cause cancer in humans at some level."*[17]

Therefore, when you see nitrite as a preservative in canned meat, bacon, ham, sausages, or hot dogs, just minimize your intake, if you can.

In addition, do you know that some of your favorite hot dogs could be made out of *"Ground Up Lips, Snouts, Spleens, Tongues, Throats, and Other Variety Meats."*[18]

Nitrite is commonly found in the following:

- Bacons
- Canned meat
- Hams (beef, chicken, pork, or turkey)
- Hot dogs
- Sausages (various kinds of meat)

Suggestion: When shopping for the above food choices, try to choose those that are made with 100% natural ingredients, if available.

10) *BHT and BHA*
(Butylated Hydroxytoluene and Butylated Hydroxyanisole)

In order to hold the color and prolong flavor in food, manufacturers use BHT or BHA as preservative. Although it protects the shelf life of the food, it could actually bring harm to your innocent body.

Even though BHT and BHA are banned in England and some other countries, these preservatives are commonly found in baked goods, beer, butter, cereals, chewing gum, dehydrated potatoes, meats, shortening, and snack foods in the U.S.

According to Christine Hoza Farlow D. C., author of *"Food Additives: A Shopper's Guide To What's Safe and What's Not,"* both BHT and BHA could cause the following:[19]

- Liver and kidney damage
- Behavioral problems
- Infertility
- Weakened immune system
- Birth defects, cancer; should be avoided by infants, young children, pregnant woman, and those sensitive to aspirin.

More disturbing facts (Parents beware): BHT could also be found in big brand names' very cute (innocent and harmless looking) children's cereals and so-called adults' healthy cereals. Go for 100% organic cereals or look for those that are made with 100% natural ingredients, whenever possible.

BHT and BHA are commonly found in:

- Baked goods
- Beer
- Butter
- Cereals (including children's cereals)
- Chewing gums
- Dehydrated potatoes
- Meats
- Shortening
- Snacks

11) Artificial Color

The more attractive and colorful processed food is, the more coloring has been added to your food. Take, for example, children's cereal or adult beverages and packaged foods. Avoid giving your children food that uses artificial color whenever possible, because food coloring may cause the following:[20]

- Hay fever
- Hyperactivity in children
- Learning and visual disorders
- Nerve damage
- Skin irritation
- Upset stomach
- Tumors in lab animals

For adults, coloring will not help you grow healthier either. Why add more chemicals to your body unnecessarily? Go for organic or natural food color products whenever you can; or at least choose products that have less artificial color added. Avoid products that are unnaturally colorful and attractive.

Coloring is commonly found in processed foods:

- Toothpaste (including children's toothpaste)
- Cereals
- Chips
- Candies
- Cheese
- Desserts

- Icing
- Meat
- Fruit or salty snacks
- Soft drinks
- Canned foods
- Frozen foods
- Packaged foods

12) Aspartame Anyone?

If you are concerned with bad breath after you eat, instead of being convinced by many gum advertisers to chew their Aspartame (so-called fat and sugar free) and BHT (food preservative) gum, why not use the natural way? Chew on natural raw fennel seeds to get healthier results.

Try this: Chew 10 – 15 tiny fennel seeds and you will get the minty taste you want. Furthermore, people from South Asia believe that it will help with digestion as well. If you are looking to add a little sweetness to the minty fennel seeds, many Indian or Mediterranean grocery stores do carry sugar-coated fennel seeds.

We know that sugar isn't good for you, so how do you use them responsibly? Just take 3-5 tiny sugar-coated fennel seeds and mix them with 10 – 15 plain fennel seeds. Chew them together and they will give you the sweetness and minty taste that is similar to gum.[21],[22]

Common side effects – Aspartame may cause:

- Fatigue
- Irritability
- Headache
- Depression
- Anxiety
- Vision problems
- Dizziness
- Memory loss
- Hyperactivity
- Migraine
- Aggression & Insomnia
- Brain damage
- Central nervous system disturbances

In addition, if you have joint problems or arthritis, you may want to avoid it whenever possible.

Aspartame is commonly found in the following:

- Sugar-free candies
- Diet or Sugar-free desserts
- Sugar-free chewing gum
- Diet or Sugar-free ice-cream
- Diet or Sugar-free sodas
- Diet or Sugar-free yogurt
- Other "Diet" or "Sugar Free" products

Remember the key words: Minimize it or cut it out whenever you can!

13) Sulfites

Sulfites can come in various forms, such as:[23]

- Potassium metabisulfite
- Potassium sulfite
- Sodium bisulfite
- Sodium hydrosulfite
- Sodium sulfite
- Sodium metabisulfite
- Sulfur dioxide or sulfuric acid.

"Sulfites" are another great food preserver; but they won't preserve your body.

Although, they have been banned from use to preserve fresh fruits and vegetables, sufites may still be added in the following food categories:[24] Based on book by Debby Anglesey.

- Dried fruits
- Wine, beer
- Mayonnaise, salad dressings
- Dairy products
- Processed cheese spread, filled crackers
- Hot dogs, sausages, bacon
- Pickles, olive, sauerkraut
- Fruit juice (bottled or frozen)
- Soft drinks
- Flour tortillas, crackers, cookies
- Bottled lemon juice

- Canned vegetables
- Pickled products – onions, relish or pickles
- Tomato puree, paste or stewed
- Flaked coconut
- Potato chips, dehydrated or frozen potatoes
- Gelatin, jams or jellies

Other common side effects caused by sulfites are:

- Asthma trigger
- Backache
- Bronchial spasms
- Burning back and muscles
- Chills or feeling cold
- Diarrhea
- Dull eyes
- Gastric distress
- Headache (Migraines)
- Inflammation of mouth's mucous membranes and mouth lesions
- Itchy skin.
- Teeth on edge, sensitive
- Increase salivation

Minimize it whenever you can! Choose alternative products that do not contain sulfites.

14) Pesticides

What is a pesticide?

A pesticide is a substance that is used for preventing, repelling, or destroying pests. Pesticides are commonly used in plantations and farms to remove weeds, insects, rats, and other unwelcome plants and animals. Think about it, if these chemicals are powerful enough to kill insects and pests, they can probably destroy some good cells in your body as well. Although evidence of the side effects due to the consumption of pesticide through food is getting stronger every day, it is wise not to sacrifice your body or your children's to be a part of the research.

Potential side effects:[25]

- Birth defects
- Cancer
- Nerve damage
- Weakened immune system

"Why Should You Care About Pesticides?"

> *"There is growing consensus in the scientific community that small doses of pesticides and other chemicals can adversely affect people, especially during vulnerable periods of fetal development and childhood when exposures can have long lasting effects. Because the toxic effects of pesticides are worrisome, not well understood, or in some cases completely unstudied, shoppers are wise to minimize exposure to pesticides whenever possible."[26]*

To minimize your consumption of pesticides from food, it is important for you to choose organic, or at least 100% natural food over non-organic ones; whenever available or possible.

3
Why Organic?

In general, any food that is labeled "Organic," must be produced without artificial fertilizers, synthetic pesticides, bioengineering, or radiation (used to kill bacteria). Prior to labeling a product as "Organic," a government-approved certifier must first inspect the farm and ensure that the farmer adheres to specific standards that are regulated by the USDA (United States Department of Agriculture).

Furthermore, organic crops are produced with earth-friendly processes using renewable resources to protect the environment for our future generations. Just as important, animals on organic farms are raised without antibiotics, genetic modification, or growth hormones.

Is organic food really more expensive than regular food?

Yes, by comparing the price of organic food to "regular" food, in general, you will see a price difference of 30– 50% or more. . . in the beginning. But when you take a minute to think of the side effects of the 14 Things to minimize in our foods (such as, Artificial Food Colorings, BHT and BHA or Other Chemical Preservatives, MSG, Aspartame, and Pesticides), organic foods may not seem expensive after all. The bottom line is:

1) Choose organic foods if available and possible.
2) Wash all fresh fruits and vegetables thoroughly before eating or cooking.

You could try the following, especially for non-organic fresh fruits and vegetables:

- Squeeze half a lime or lemon into clean water and soak your fruits or vegetables for five minutes. Then wash or scrub your fresh fruits and vegetables thoroughly before eating or cooking.

Alternatives:
Try exploring your local Mom and Pop grocery stores. Some of them have already started carrying fresh and packaged organic foods. If you are lucky, those stores may price their organic foods very competitively with their conventional foods. As for your favorite chain grocery stores, they may offer discounts on different organic items on a weekly or bi-weekly basis.

Cut down on your junk food purchases and save your money for organic food.

If you are eating out, save the money you were spending on soft drinks and desserts, and use it for organic foods instead. At least three positive things can happen if you substitute soda with water and cut down on desserts:

You will have saved enough money to buy organic foods.
You can cut down on sugar, salt, MSG, saturated fat, and trans fats, naturally. Your self-esteem and confidence will go up because you are able to control your thoughts and resist those unhealthy foods' temptations.

4
33 Helpful Tips:

1) Best Substitutes

Use or Choose:
- Organic sugar **over** table or regular sugar
- 100% whole wheat or whole grain flour **over** any kind of enriched flour
- Brown rice **over** white rice
- Organic fruits and vegetables **over** non-organic ones. If only conventional fruits and vegetables are available, scrub and wash them thoroughly before eating or cooking; I'm doing that too!
- Organic whole grain bread or 100% whole wheat bread **over** any enriched flour bread
- Organic pasta or 100% natural whole grain pasta **over** regular pasta
- Organic lean meat or 100% natural lean meat **over** meat with hormones or antibiotics
- Organic pasta sauce or 100% natural pasta sauce **over** regular pasta sauce
- Distilled, purified, or filtered water **over** soda or coffee
- Blended fresh fruit juice or squeezed juice **over** boxed or canned juice
- Filtered room temperature to very warm water **over** cold or ice water
- 100% pure olive oil **over** other kinds of vegetable or hydrogenated oils
- Sleep at least 8 hours or close to 8 hours per night **over** caffeine, energy pills, or drinks

Good Rule of Thumb:

- Minimize your intake of unhealthy foods

- Choose organic or 100% natural ingredients over artificial ingredients

2) *Three Other Things That Are Not Good For You:*

- **Nicotine**
- **Alcohol**
- **Illegal Drugs**

Common side effects:
- Lung cancer
- High blood pressure
- Kidney problems
- Heart attack
- Drunk driving
- Parents' nicotine and alcohol habits are one of the major causes of their children's gateway to nicotine and alcohol addiction. These substances also open the doors to illegal drugs
- Fatal accidents and
- The list goes on and on...

Yes, some researchers have found that alcohol may be helpful to the body. If you know the limit suggested by the researchers, and you can limit your intake to that level, that's your choice! Otherwise, avoid if at all possible.

We all know that nicotine, alcohol, and illegal drugs do more harm to our innocent bodies than good.

"By eliminating bad habits of over-eating, drinking [alcohol] too much, smoking, or using harmful drugs and replacing them with healthy habits, we can prevent the causes of deadly disease."[27] — *W. Clement Stone*

3) Question

Should I Stop Eating All My Favorite Junk Food Right Away?

Going cold turkey is not recommended unless your doctor advises it. Why? Since it probably took a long time for you to build up your poor eating habits, you should give yourself a little time to cut down on junk food, one step at a time.

Let's fill your stomach with more healthy foods first and gradually phase out those unhealthy foods. Instead of eating 80% junk food and 20% healthy foods every day, let's reverse it gradually and work healthy foods into your system.

The space in your stomach has a limit unless you choose to overeat and over-stretch it. If you calm your mind down and listen to your Inner Healthy Voice (Chapter 7), you should become aware of the signal from your body that says you are full. Have you ever noticed that sometimes you can hear your Inner Voice saying, "If I eat another of this...I will be so... full?" This is the sign of your Inner Healthy Voice urging you to stop eating. But if you let your Inner Junky Voice dictate your eating habits, it will be hard for you to lose weight and get healthy.

4) Don't Beat Yourself Up...

What if your weight goes down a few pounds and goes back up a couple of pounds?

This is very normal. This book is about changing bad habits, not a quick fix. Bad habits take time to break. If you gain a couple of pounds back, DO NOT WORRY!!!

Just go back and think of when, how, and what you have eaten for the past three meals. You will be able to figure out where your extra pounds have come from.

Gaining that couple of pounds back couldn't have really been that easy. You must have substituted soda, concentrated juice, or creamy sugar coffee for water; fried food for steamed or grilled food; overeaten; eaten late at night; or slept after a meal.

The fun thing about MIND YOUR OWN WELLNESS is that it allows you to go back and forth to figure out how to lose your weight faster and, why, how, or what you did to gain it back. The choices are yours because you are now the CEO of your body and your main job is to eat 80% healthier food and leave 20% maximum for entertainment or junk food.

5) Who Is In control – You Or The Food?

Celebrations, graduations, parties, a meeting with an old friend, family gatherings, just wanting to reward yourself for no reason, or wanting a break is OK! Just remember to at least use the White Belt's Success Formula (Chapter 16) so that you do not fall back into the stress cycle and start eating all you want again.

The power of water: Having 10–20% of the volume of your stomach full of water will naturally limit your junk food intake to only 80–90%. You will feel full quicker without having to eat up 100% of the junk food portion like you've done in the past. *Now,* when your Inner Healthy Voice signals you to stop, do not be tempted to take another bite.

Suggestion:

If you feel sick after your party or take-a-break day, recall the kinds of food that made you sick. More often than not, the food that you have eaten belongs to the 14 Things (Chapter 2) that you should minimize. Eat less of those! Reassure yourself that, "I'm in control, not the food."

6) Responsibilities

Parenting tips

Are you really doing the best for your kids? Saving money or wealth for your kids is great, however, it is not as good as being *there* for them, especially when your kids are between the ages of 0 and 18. Children need a lot of physical and mental support, as well as love from parents. They need quantity and quality time to guide them through good and bad times.

This book will set a great example for them, and being there for them is absolutely priceless. It is good to set your basic goal to at least MIND YOUR OWN WELLNESS for your family. Why give your life away prematurely to unhealthy food or overeating habits?

It is good to guide your loved ones toward the happy goal of staying healthy. These are some of the trickle-down effects:

- When you start eating right, you will be able to influence your loved ones to follow in your footsteps through your positive energy. This is especially true with children!

- If you are overweight or have poor eating habits, it will be hard for your kids *not* to follow your poor eating habits. *"Children don't do as you say, they do as you do."* Eat light and healthy, and your children will enjoy the positive effects of your role modeling. And *their* children will follow in their footsteps. You will leave a lasting legacy!

- Life will be less stressful if everyone in your family is healthy. Why would you choose to have poor eating habits that turn you into a sick person who isn't 100% there for your family?

Listen to your Inner Healthy Voice, focus on healthier food choices and you will be on your way to MIND YOUR OWN WELLNESS. After all, staying healthy is not as hard as you thought. It is a matter of getting used to and following through with just ONE MAIN ACTION – EAT LESS UNHEALTHY FOOD!

7) Parenting Tips II

The food or treats that taste the best for your kids could be harmful to their bodies. If you routinely let your children eat foods that contain the 14 Things that you should minimize, it could potentially speed up their health problems. Start by gradually switching their unhealthy habits to the better ones as soon as you can.

8) How do you know if you have overeaten?

Signs of overeating:

- Shortness of breath or shallow breathing
- Stiff neck
- Feeling tired after eating; feeling like sleeping
- Body discomfort
- Feeling frustrated or angry for no good reason
- Stress
- Moodiness
- Bloating
- Craving for more salty snacks or sweet desserts, even when you are full

9) Smart Eating Habits

Filling your stomach with at least 80% healthy food will help you create the good eating habit of not wanting junk food. Have you noticed that food tastes best when you are extremely hungry? Your favorite junk food does not taste as good when you are so full that you really could not take another bite! Gradually, your craving for junk food will be reduced and your Inner Junky Voice (Chapter 7) will no longer be in charge.

Caution: If you reverse the strategy and start eating 80% unhealthy food first and leave the rest for healthy food, your desire for healthier food will be reduced gradually. Eventually, you may be filling yourself up with more than 80% junk and no longer like the food that is good for your heart. But don't worry – every day is a new chance to put on the Color Belt (Chapter 16) that is right for you!

10) Free Sugar Refills Anyone? Is it Worth It?

Say "NO" To Free Sugar Refills:

Every time you drink a free sugar-water refill, it's like you are driving your body directly to the health-challenged HIGHWAY. Sugar gets into your system quickly and weakens your immune system in no time. Worst of all, the more sugar you consume, the more you crave it. Natural sugar from fruits and vegetables are better, *and* they come with fiber and vitamins.

Imagine that you have just had a full 16oz. soda (the equivalent of approximately 45 grams of sugar). Why do you need another 45 grams of sugar in one meal? Train yourself to see sugar from processed foods and drinks as FAT; NOT FAT FREE! Any amount of sugar that you consume will be turned into fat if your body cannot burn it off in a quick amount of time.

11) *Buffet, Buffet All The Way!*

Is it worth it? How much can you gain out of buffets? If you could eat twice or three times as much, do you actually come out ahead? On the surface, it is worth it, to eat more than you paid for. But realistically, you are gaining weight by eating two or three times as much as you need. Unfortunately, the gain is never a profit in your pocket. It is in pounds on the scale.

It will be more fun and pleasurable if your goal is to explore different kinds of food that buffet restaurants offer, or to give yourself a break from your routine meals without overeating. The *good* thing about buffets is that they normally offer a choice of fresh fruits and vegetables. Eat that first! And remember, a good strategy for buffet eating is to use at least the White Belt's Success Formula in Chapter 16.

12) *Weigh Yourself Only Once Or Twice A Week In The Morning!*

Let it be natural. Be aware not to overeat and substitute soda with water and gradually add more fresh fruits and vegetables into your diet. Your weight will come down steadily, one pound at a time. Weigh yourself first thing in the morning only! How you feel in your clothes, and how much energy you have, is a better indicator of your health than what the scale tells you. Weighing yourself everyday or after every meal is likely to add more stress to your life.

13) *How Do We Usually Eat When We Are Very Hungry And In A Hurry?*

Like a food vampire, many busy people with lots of responsibilities take very few bites and swallow food very quickly. Whenever we are rushing, we have the tendency to forget to chew our food well before we swallow. Yes, we may save a few minutes, but we are actually adding extra burdens to our stomach.

The larger the chunk of food that we swallow, the longer and harder it will take to digest. When we eat in a hurry, it increases the chance of overeating because we will not feel full as quickly. By the time we feel full, we have already eaten more than we need. Indigestion often comes along and is followed by tiredness, headache, and stomach discomfort. Even if you think you need to rush through a meal, how far ahead will you be if you feel awful afterwards? Hydrate yourself with 1 glass of water first, and remind yourself this: *"Whenever I am very hungry and in a hurry, I really need to slow down and chew my food well."*

14) Cravings:

If your craving is so bad that you can't resist junk food after dinner, do this:

1. Drink two full glasses of water
2. Eat one portion of fresh fruit (apple, banana, grapes, or orange)
3. Then eat your junk food

Typically, after you finish your two portions of water and one portion of fresh fruit, your craving for junk food will be reduced, because your stomach is now filled with the really good stuff instead of junk food. Even if you still crave for junk food, the portion of junk that you will eat will be limited because you are already full! Good Job!

15) *The Good, The Bad, And The Ugly Habits To Manage STRESS...*

The Good — When stress hits, the person with good habits will choose to eat light and go for an hour-long workout to recharge the body with oxygen and the natural high energy that comes from exercise.

The Bad — When stress appears, the person will listen to the Inner Junky Voice for advice, "Eat that cheesecake or bag of chips so that you can have a sense of control and it will make you feel good. Or, go for a buffet lunch/dinner so that you can forget about the stressful situation."

The Ugly — Combine the Bad with sleep after overeating and you are sure to gain weight fast and double your stress.

Which kinds of habits do you have?

Train yourself to build a new habit. When stress arrives, use the Red or Black Belt's Success Formula in Chapter 16 to help you manage your situation. With the Red or Black Belt's Success Formula, you will find that (after eating) you can concentrate better and handle any stressful situation well. Using junk food to reduce stress will only worsen your situation and it is only temporary relief. It only lasts for the moment you are eating. Once you have finished all your junk food, your stress will come right back.

Not only have you not reduced your stress, you have just added more burden to your body. Because unhealthy foods are high in sugar, salt, and fat - they actually take away energy that your body needs to burn fat, instead of giving you the energy to be productive at work.

16) Ways Of Getting Stressed

Causes: External (beyond your control) and Internal (self-generated)

Your choices: Get stressed or find a solution!

You aren't overweight for no reason at all. Many of us have gotten this way because we have forgotten or never learned the effective and positive ways to handle our stress. Do these unhealthy ways of dealing with stress keep you from living your life the way you want to?

- Do you focus on the past and continue to lock into the stress mode?
- Do you blame others or yourself for the situation?
- Do you keep thinking of the "What Ifs" and not moving forward to find solutions?
- Do you do nothing, literally nothing, and just sit there and keep thinking about the past?
- Do you have too much free time?
- Do you take shallower and shallower breaths until you've almost forgotten to breathe?
- Do you stand like a hunch-back with your back curved instead of confident and straight?
- Have you subconsciously lost the smile on your face, and have you started to frown?
- Do you get headaches and feel more stressed than ever?
- Do you automatically go for "Junk Food Favorites" like ice cream, chocolate, chips, fries, cookies, and soda?
- Once you are through with your feel-good junk food, do you become more stressed than ever because you have just added more guilt to your life?
- Do you sleep or sit and watch TV and hope that the situation will get better by itself?

- Do you take diet pills to try to lose the weight that you have just gained? Remember, the side effects of the pills may make you feel worse.
- Do you start to get impatient or mean with other innocent people such as family members, friends, or the public? What goes around will come around — when you are mean to people, it normally finds a way to come back to haunt you.
- Is your life going from bad to worse because of all of the above?

17) Potential Solutions For Stress

Once you feel stressed, give yourself a TIME-OUT. Think as Napoleon Hill said in his CDs' *Think and Grow Rich*, *"No circumstance in your life can make you feel a certain way, unless you and only you allow it to happen."*[28] Do the following:

- Put on a smile, not a frown.
- Sit or stand up with an upright posture.
- Take a few deep breaths and continue with your deep breathing exercises. Or use the 5-5-10 breathing exercise to help you. (Chapter 12)
- Eat light and take a 10–15 minute walk after you eat. Remember, when stress hits, eat light. (Drink a glass of water or hot green tea, eat an apple or orange, or snack on a fresh sweet carrot stick; instead of soda, potato chips, or chocolate).
- Focus solely on the present and future. What are the things that you can do to improve the situation. Think of the solutions, *not* problems.

- If it is not too late to do something about the stressful situation, do it now or plan it out in writing so that you do not forget.
- If there is nothing you can do about the stress and you know it is your mistake, take responsibility and learn from it; don't repeat it again.
- If it is not your mistake, think of what you might be able to learn from others' mistakes so that it does not happen to you in the future.
- If someone lies to you, don't get mad at the person for lying. Just tell yourself that it is useful information that this person lies a lot, and watch out in the future. Act accordingly! If somebody makes a mess, that somebody gets to clean it up! If people learn that you don't get EMOTIONAL every time something bad happens, if they see that you get PAST THAT and either act on it or use it as good information, THAT'S what helps!.
- Take life as a fun learning process. There is always something for you to learn in every situation. The only question is: Will you choose to take life as a fun and enjoyable learning process, or will you choose to turn every challenge in your life into stressful situations. THE CHOICE IS ABSOLUTELY YOURS.

18) Night Or After-Dinner Strategy

What happens if you are still hungry after dinner?
Answer: Drink an 8-ounce cup of water.

What if you are really, really feeling hungry after dinner or late at night?

Solution: Drink another 8-ounce cup of water. Then focus on the end result of feeling energetic and light the next morning, instead of feeling tired and heavy.

When you are drinking just water, you have to pay careful attention to your Inner Junky Voice, because it will start to communicate, beg, demand, and influence you to give up your staying- healthy goal. It may start to talk to you in the following ways:

"Life sucks if I cannot eat what I want, when I want it!"
"It is no fun if I have to control this, control that!"
"Just eat it, what the heck!"
"Just a little junk food won't hurt!"

If you're not careful, the Inner Junky Voice will keep nagging until you fall into its trap.

Instead, think about the reasons you are still hungry after dinner:

1) Old bad habits.
2) Staying up too late. Sometimes you need sleep, not food!
3) You are stuck to your TV for hours and you let those unhealthy food advertisements adversely influence your staying-healthy goals!
4) Excuses!

Take control; do not let your Inner Junky Voice affect your decision to stay healthy and well. When morning comes around, you will be so glad that you managed to stay in control and did not eat junk food after dinner. If you happen to give in and eat that junk, take advantage of the situation and make mental notes of how that particular junk food affects your sleep, energy, and emotion, the next morning. Don't make the same mistake again. Avoid junk food after dinner, whenever possible.

19) Late At Night

Have you ever noticed what happens to your stomach from about 10:00 at night until about 2:00 in the morning?

Do you usually feel like eating something during that period? Everyone has heard of midnight snacks! Have you also noticed the change in advertisements on TV around that time? They are for deep-fried meals, chocolate, delicious burgers, sausage, and egg meals. They start to pop out more to tell you what to eat for breakfast, lunch, and dinner for tomorrow.

Once you are aware of what those advertisers are doing to your thoughts, it will be harder for your Inner Junky Voice to play with what you will be eating tomorrow. You will have control over what is really good and healthy for you the next day. Just stick to your game plan to eat right, unless it is your take-a-break day.

If you really want to stay healthy, you can. Be patient and persistent and you will soon feel a change. You will feel lighter and breath deeper, move faster, and your confidence level will increase. Before you know it, you will be amazed by the changes that your new choices have made in your life.

20) Specific Suggestion For Change

Always be open to listening to your Inner Healthy Voice (Chapter 7).

Your hunger after a full dinner has to do with your old habits. There is room for a change!

Say to yourself, "There is really no need for me to eat anything after dinner except water. At most, I can be healthy with a slice of toast, or one portion of fresh fruit or vegetable."

Focus on the following sentence:

"By replacing junk food after dinner with water, my health conditions will improve drastically, I will feel lighter and more energetic the next morning. Nice fresh delicious water will help cleanse my body instead of adding burdens to my health."

21) Quick Fix = Quick Comeback

Quick fixes are often temporary! They usually do not last. Approximately 90% of all adults in America who went on a diet gained their weight back soon after their diet program was over, and then some. Why? Because, if you do not train yourself to stop putting bad food into your mouth, even though you look great due to the quick-fix diet medicine, surgery, or starvation-diet programs, your health could potentially suffer and the slimming effect could only be short term. In addition, many diet pills come with FREE side effects too. At least one diet product could cause hair loss on the head and hair growth on the face when one is not careful and overuses it!

22) The Fact

Everyone wants good health, either consciously or sub-consciously. And we know a healthy body will bring more joy and less stress to life. Through praying and other forms of meditation and request, good health will always make us feel the best.

Simply stated: Good eating habits will bring good health. Poor eating habits will lead to poor health, no matter how sincere you are with your prayer. Everything that you eat and drink will either help or deteriorate your health. You can spend 24 hours a day praying for good health; but, if your daily food consists of only unhealthy foods, your health will not be good. There is no way out!

Since you will soon be equipped with the cool 5 Color Belts' Success Formulas in Chapter 16, it is all up to you how healthy you want yourself to be. In combination with your prayers, this book can lead you to better health.

23) Blending Versus Juicing - Is There A difference?

It all depends on how you do it. In case you are not aware, the skins of many fruits and root vegetables are the main source of their fiber and antioxidants. If you remove them prior to eating, you are actually taking away the essential fiber that is good for your digestive system. Therefore, it is important to wash your fruits and vegetable thoroughly before eating.

If you blend organic apples or pears with their skin, the amount of fiber you will get from the fruits will be maximized. Although the texture of the blended juice is coarser than juice from the juicer, you are getting the natural fiber that will help you digest better and keep your digestive system in good working order.

A juice machine is good too, but juicers tend to hold back a portion of fiber (usually the skin of the fruits) in the filters.

24) What About Salad?

Salad is great. You can replace the one or two portions of salad with a portion or two of fresh fruits if you like. However, if you want dressing, you need to read the label. By adding 2 to 4 tablespoons of dressing to your salad, you can easily add 9 to 18 grams of fat and 7 to 14 grams of sugar into your body.

If you choose to stay healthy, pay attention to the amount and the kind of dressing that you are using. Avoid dressings that contain high fat, high sodium/salt, and high sugar, whenever possible. Especially beware of those that come with MSG —

avoid them if you can. Recall your goal and remind yourself, "I choose to stay healthy and I choose to limit my dressing so I can eat right and feel great."

25) Ice Water, Room Temperature Water, Or Very Warm Drinking Water – Is There A Difference?

On the surface, it might not seem to matter. After all, cold or hot water is just water. Right? Think and see if the following make sense to you.

When I was a kid, I thought that cold water was better for me because it helped cool me down right away, especially when the weather was hot. Although my Dad and Mom often deterred me from drinking ice-cold water or eating ice cream, I continued to drink ice-cold water and eat ice cream as much as I could when my parents were not with me. For years, I would not listen to their advice until I took up martial arts and got bruises, bumps, and sprains. After visiting several Chinese Physicians for different injuries, they all said the same thing, "Avoid ice or cold water and ice cream too!" "Why?" I asked. "Because ice or cold water and ice cream, will slow down your blood circulation and it will take longer for your injuries to heal. Worst of all, it will cause 'Rheumatism' when you get older."

What is rheumatism? Rheumatism comes in different forms. The kind of rheumatism that my Chinese Physicians talked about is similar to arthritis, with joint pains or other sharp pains coming back from old injuries or overuse. How?

It could potentially turn you into an automatic weather forecasting machine. For example, if you are suffering from minor rheumatism, you will be able to tell when a storm is coming a couple of hours prior to the storm because your past injuries will start giving you pain. Most people, in general, will treat their symptoms as if they have arthritis. They will take pain-relief pills to ease their symptoms while they continue to drink their favorite ice water, soda with ice, or eat ice cream routinely. They will wonder why their arthritis is going from bad to worse! As for severe rheumatic sufferers, their natural forecasting system is far more accurate. They can feel the acute rheumatic pains (especially if they have previous broken bone injuries) many hours before the storm or rain arrives. Ouch!

Fortunately, as dumb as I was for not listening to my Dad and Mom's advice (just because they were not physicians), I did listen to the Chinese physicians and I finally stopped wondering why my parents wanted me to avoid drinking too much ice or cold water – ice cream included. My parents simply did not want me to suffer in the future. Years later, I found out why Dad was more firm than Mom about not wanting me to drink ice or cold water and eat too much ice cream. It was because my Dad actually got it from experience. He was in martial arts too and he had dealt with rheumatism before.

As with my other recommendations, you do not have to totally cut out your ice water or ice cream. Just minimize it, if possible.

If the above is not convincing enough, think of the following:

Imagine your body as a car engine. Why is it best for you to warm it up before you drive it, especially during SUB ZERO winters? Circulation! You need to heat up your car engine in order to prolong the life of your engine and prevent it from breaking down too soon. Similarly, your body temperature is always heated up at +/-37° C or +/- 98.6 °F when you are feeling well. Drinking ice-cold water or eating ice cream regularly is like pouring gallons of ice water on top of a heated car engine. It will lower your engine's temperature or slow it down suddenly.

Day in and day out, if you do this to your car engine, it will break down prematurely. The breaking down of the engine is like rheumatism in humans.

If you are not worried about rheumatism, drink ice water, ice-cold soda, and eat ice cream, just like you did before. However, if you would like to minimize your chance of getting rheumatism, cut it down. By far, I have not come across any Star Rheumatism Club Member who thinks that having rheumatism is a fun and pleasurable process. Sometimes the pain also hits Rheumatic Members during their sleep too, just because storms are coming. Ouch! Ouch! Double Ouch!

26) Power Of Organic Apple Cider Vinegar

Honestly, I do not like the smell of it at first, because I simply do not like vinegar. However, once I acquired the taste, it tastes a little like lemonade.

Start by adding one teaspoon of organic apple cider vinegar to half a glass of water (4oz) and drink it - add a little honey if necessary. Once you are used to the taste, you could increase to one tablespoon of organic apple cider vinegar to an 8oz glass of water.

When do I drink it? You could drink it once after lunch and once after dinner. It is especially helpful to drink it whenever you overeat, or after eating an unhealthy oily meal. Besides helping with digestion, the following are just some of Organic Apple Cider Vinegar's benefits:[29]

- *Helps remove artery plaque and body toxins*
- *Helps fight germs, viruses, and bacteria naturally*
- *Helps normalize urine pH, relieving frequent urge to urinate*
- *Helps relieve sore throats*
- *Helps detox the body so sinus, asthma, and flu sufferers can breathe easier and more normally*

- *Helps banish acne, soothes burns and sunburns*
- *Helps fight arthritis and removes crystals and toxins from joints, tissues, organs and entire body*
- *Helps control and normalize body weight*

For full details about the benefits of Organic Apple Cider Vinegar, read *Bragg's Apple Cider Vinegar* by Paul C. Bragg, N.D., Ph.D. and Patricia Bragg, N.D., Ph.D.

27) Positive Thoughts

How much are you worth? When you are at the lowest point in life, you might think you are worthless. However, if a millionaire wants to pay you $1 million dollars for your heart, would you sell it to the millionaire? No! Take good care of your body so that it can take good care of you!

28) Know Your Goal (Stay Healthy) And Stick To It!

"If There Is A Will, There Is A Way."

As you follow the recommendations in this book, recognize that your Inner Junky Voice, advertisements, and easily available junk foods are always trying to move you away from your healthy goal. Watch out for your Inner Junky Voice that tries to persuade you to eat more unhealthy food than you need. The voice might say something like:

- "I really must eat this smooth creamy chocolate"
- "I will go on strict diet after I eat this Monster Double Chocolate Cheese Cake"
- "Come on, it is a double cheese burger – It is so delicious and it is a deluxe!"
- "Just eat it; I will never be healthy anyway"
- "It is free, go ahead and eat it"

- "Yum! Yum! Super Deep Fried Crispy Chicken – Buy four pieces, get four pieces free - Today only!"
- "If I don't eat it now, I may die tomorrow."

When you hear these things, try these strategies for sticking to your goal:

- Avoid the temptation — Say to your Inner Junky Voices, "I don't want it!"
- Procrastinate — Wait till tomorrow for that junk food.
- If worse comes to worse, minimize the bad food — Instead of buying a large bag of chips, buy the smallest bag available.

29) Being Present

Pay attention to who is controlling your body.

If your Inner Healthy Voice is in charge, you are in good shape! If your Inner Junky Voice is in control, you are probably out of shape.

Slow down when you eat. Give yourself a chance to enjoy the food you are eating. Once you slow down, you will be able to taste your food better. Especially when you are eating desserts or treats, you will suddenly feel the super sweet or salty taste you are just about to swallow.

If you keep your awareness high enough, you will also be able to feel that the inside of your mouth and your teeth are coated with oil or lard when you are eating deep fried food. At this time, your Inner Healthy Voice will clue you stop eating sooner. And, this is the power of being present. It will help you to choose to reduce your sugar, salt, and oil intake consciously.

However, if you choose to continue to finish up the entire bowl of ice cream, three pieces of deep fried chicken, and a large side order of mashed potato because of your past habits (always eating up all unhealthy food), then you have to bear with the consequences — probably gaining a few more pounds every month.

30) Pay Attention, Observe, Be Aware

Take a look at your plate after you finish your meal. Notice that when you order a healthier meal such as baked fish, steamed vegetables, and the like, washing dishes is easier to do! But when you order deep fried or cheesy food, after you finish your meal, the leftover residue is often very sticky, greasy, and harder to clean. In addition, try putting a few pieces of ice from your soda on your greasy plate and see what happens. The leftover grease or oil will harden and turn into saturated fat almost instantly.

Can you imagine the same thing happening inside your stomach?

If it is going to take a longer time for you to wash off that grease from your plate, that same grease will stay in your stomach longer and it will require great efforts for your stomach to digest!

31) Beware Of Junk Food - On Sale!

Imagine you are at the grocery store and see a sign for a super sale on junk food. Remember that it might look like a good deal, but buying these foods will have a negative effect on your health. For example:

- Now bigger: 30% more unhealthy food for the same price! **True meaning:** It is time to put on more weight.
- Buy 1 get 1 half off! **True meaning:** Start blocking your arteries!
- Buy 2 bags of chips for the price of 1! **True meaning:** Since your heart is still pumping, let's weaken it!
- Holiday Special – Buy this junk, get that junk free! **True meaning:** It is the end of the year; let us increase our weight first before the next year comes!
- 50% off for the last 2 days! **True meaning:** You have 2 days left to think about bringing forward your heart operation's date!
- Buy 1 bag of junk food, get 1 free! **True meaning:** Speed up your pains twice as fast!

Buying junk food on sale basically means adding fat to your body and adding emotional pain to your life. Let us face the facts! The more junk food you buy, the more you or your family will eat it. Avoid junk food sales and start taking control of your health. Minimize your junk food intake if possible or buy the smallest size available.

32) Switch Your Focus

The more you think of the junk food that you love to eat, the more it will become irresistible. That is what advertisements do. They could change your state of mind from feeling fine to feeling hungry in 30 seconds. And if you sit in front of your TV long enough, the same advertisement or other delicious food advertisements will hit your brain again and again until you suddenly feel hungry again. You will start reaching out for junk food or start calling for food delivery even though you just had dinner a couple of hours ago.

What kinds of food do you think you would eat after you were consciously or subconsciously trapped by TV advertisements? JUNK FOOD!!! Something sweet, salty, or oily!!!

The next time you are hit by those junk food advertisements, switch your focus and remind yourself, "Those are the kinds of foods that cause body pain and make you drift away from being healthy." If you really think that you need to eat something, drink a glass of water or procrastinate till tomorrow's lunch or your Take-A-Break day (Chapter 15). You already know that eating junk food prior to sleeping is the surest way to make your health deteriorate physically and mentally; not to mention, you will also be wasting your money on junk food and diet pills.

33) Think! Unhealthy Food = Pain

If you know that something you are about to put into your mouth will bring pain to your life, why do you eat it? Just because it tastes good or you are convinced by the advertisements?

The following is a great Pain and Pleasure strategy that I've learned from The Great Motivator Anthony Robbins:

How to control your mind:

The next time you see junk food, train your mind to associate it with pain and speeding up health problems. The more you train yourself to link junk food with pain or disease, the sooner you will be able to decode those junk food advertisements and listen less to your Inner Junky Voice (Chapter 7). Just a reminder: Junk food should not be the main dish of every meal.

In order to get more pleasure out of your life, simply eat more plant-based (healthier) food.

Think: Unhealthy Food = Pain!

Think: Healthy Food = Pleasure!

If you choose to have a better life, eat healthier food and minimize your junk food intake. Whenever you see fresh fruits and vegetables, associate them with pleasure and healthier life.

Always remind yourself that you are in full control over your food choices. Have faith—You can do it!

5
Face The Facts

Face the facts, know where you are now, and focus all your attention on where you are heading! The past is gone! The present is now and the future is where you want to be. The present is the only place you can make a positive difference to your life.

Once you know where you are at, the goal will be to work backward into the BMI chart, one step at a time. Don't panic if you are overweight (BMI greater than 25 and less than 30) or obese (BMI greater than 30). As long as you are willing to put this book into use and take action with faith, you will be able to get yourself back on track.

No matter what your BMI is, you are certainly not alone — millions of adults in America are overweight or obese. Me too! Was on the same boat for 20 years.

What is your current BMI (Body Mass Index)?

Use these steps to determine your current BMI.

1. Measure your height in inches or feet while standing on bare feet
2. Weigh yourself first thing in the morning
3. Check the chart to determine your current BMI
4. Record the result with the date: BMI_____ Date:_____

Use this chart only as a general guideline. If you have a bigger head (like me), broader than normal shoulders, bigger muscles, or heavy or big bones, then your natural weight is probably 1 – 5 pounds heavier than normal. Just set a simple goal: "Any unwanted pounds that you managed to get rid of for good, is awesome."

Make sure that you confirm your BMI with your doctor and ask if this program is good for you. If your Doctor gives you an OK to proceed, put this book to work!

For Example: If *Height = 6 foot*; *Weight = 206 pounds*; Then _BMI is 28_ (Currently Overweight)

(See next page)

	Normal						Overweight					Obese		
BMI	19	20	21	22	23	24	25	26	27	28	29	30	35	40
Height							Weight (lb)							
4'10"	91	96	100	105	110	115	119	124	129	134	138	143	167	191
4'11"	94	99	104	109	114	119	124	128	133	138	143	148	173	198
5'	97	102	107	112	118	123	128	133	138	143	148	153	179	204
5' 1"	100	106	111	116	122	127	132	137	143	148	153	158	185	211
5' 2"	104	109	115	120	126	131	136	142	147	153	158	164	191	218
5' 3"	107	113	118	124	130	135	141	146	152	158	163	169	197	225
5' 4"	110	116	122	128	137	140	145	151	157	163	169	174	204	232
5' 5"	114	120	126	132	138	144	150	156	162	168	174	180	210	240
5' 6"	118	124	130	136	142	148	155	161	167	173	179	186	216	247
5' 7"	121	127	134	140	146	153	159	166	172	178	185	191	223	255
5' 8"	125	131	138	144	151	158	164	171	177	184	190	197	230	262
5' 9"	128	135	142	149	155	162	169	176	182	189	196	203	236	270
5' 10"	132	139	146	153	160	167	174	181	188	195	202	209	243	278
5' 11"	136	143	150	157	165	172	179	186	193	200	208	215	250	286
6'	140	147	154	162	169	177	184	191	199	206	213	221	258	294
6' 1"	144	151	159	166	174	182	189	197	204	212	219	227	265	302
6' 2"	148	155	163	171	179	186	194	202	210	218	225	233	272	311
6' 3"	152	160	168	176	184	192	200	208	216	224	232	240	279	319
6' 4"	156	164	172	180	189	197	205	213	221	230	238	246	287	328

Sources: Campbell TC, and Campbell II TM. *The China Study*. Dallas, TX: Benbella Books, Inc. 136.

Make Up Your Mind!

Decide once and for all that you are going to "MIND YOUR OWN WELLNESS" and let this book guide you to achieve your healthy goal!

"Letter Of Commitment"

I, _____,
(Your Name)

like myself. I love myself.

And I choose to

Stay Healthy.

I have FAITH that I will make it

One Step At A Time!

_____
(Your Signature)

_____
(Date)

Paste this on your mirror and read it aloud twice daily! Once in the morning and once before you sleep.

*"Copy or download this page from
www.MindYourOwnWellness.com/LOC.html
and share it with others!"*

2. Truth: Not That Easy To Be Obese

If You Think That It Is Easy To Become Obese And Stay That Way, Rather Than Healthy, Think Again...

Take a look at the amount of effort you have to make in order to stay big or get bigger. If you have managed to be obese for months or years, or you've been getting bigger each year, you already have what it takes to stay healthy (Save Money, Stay Healthy). When you look at the bottom line, you will see that it actually requires much greater energy and sacrifice physically, mentally, and financially to be big as compared to staying healthy. Give yourself a chance to experience a taste of staying healthy with MIND YOUR OWN WELLNESS.

In order to stay big or get bigger, you have to do all of the following:

Physically:

- You have to spend your money to buy all kinds of desserts.
- You have to remember to eat mostly high sugar, high salt, or oily foods even though you know for sure that in the long run, they will clog up your arteries and give you a stroke or heart attack.
- You have to make sure to overeat often.
- You have to eat late.
- You have to sleep within 1–2 hours after you eat.
- You have to constantly waste your money on junk food to satisfy your Inner Junky Voice (Chapter 7).
- You have to sit obediently and not move much after every meal.
- You have to give up your freedom to exercise.
- You have to buy new sets of clothes to accommodate your bigger and bigger sizes.

Mentally:
- You have to handle the way people look at you just because you are big, especially in any buffet restaurants.
- You have to deal with peer pressure, especially when they know that you are working on losing weight and they think that you are wasting your time.
- You have to deal with hating your own body or look.
- You may have to deal with low self-esteem and low self-confidence
- You have to deal with the stress due to overeating.
- You have to be 100% obedient to your Inner Junky Voice even though it is flushing your energy, body, and emotions down the drain.

Financially:
- You have to waste a good chunk of your hard-earned income on junk foods, such as desserts and side orders.
- You have to make sure to eat enough junk foods so that you can get constipated! Then you can spend money on pills! (Not to mention that some constipation pills do come with other side effects and then you get to spend more money to buy more pills or see your doctor to treat those side effects.)
- You have to spend more money on diet pills and drink diet sodas that contain Aspartame (could cause cancer).
- But once you are in bed, your body will have two choices: 1) You might fall asleep right away and wake up frustrated because your stomach is so bloated and you are short of breath or 2) Although you are extremely tired, once you hit the bed, you can not fall asleep because your stomach is too full and it is uncomfortable to lie down in any position. Therefore, you have to waste your money again to buy sleeping pills to help you sleep.

You really have to follow through on many of the "Have-tos" in order to stay obese. 20 years of staying obese was more than enough for me. The experience was extremely painful.

3. Are You Eating Towards The Danger Zone?

If your daily diet includes foods like the ones listed below, you could be on your way to The Danger Zone.

Breakfast:
1–2 glasses of milk (high in animal protein)
1–2 eggs (high in animal protein)
2–3 strips of bacon (high in animal protein and saturated fat)
2–3 sausage patties (high in animal protein and saturated fat)

Or milk (high in animal protein) and colorful cereals (colorings and BHT as preservatives)

1st Break-Time:
1 cup of coffee (caffeine, with cream and sugar)
1 donut (sugar and fat)
1 cigarette (smokers only - nicotine)
1 strip of sugarless gum (BHT)

Lunch Or Lunch Buffet (salt, MSG, sugar, and saturated fat):
8-24oz (1-3cups) of colored sugar soda — depending on the size of your order and whether you get free refill or not (sugar or Aspartame for Diet drinks)
1 large fries (fat)
1 double cheeseburger or fried chicken (salt and saturated fat)
Deserts: ice cream, sundaes or yummy shakes (sugar and fat)

2nd Break-Time:
1 cup of coffee (caffeine, with cream and sugar)
1 cigarette (smokers only - nicotine)
1 strip of sugarless gum (BHT)

Dinner or Buffet Dinner (salt, MSG, sugar, and saturated fat):
1-2 cups of soda (sugar) or diet soda (with Aspartame)
1-2 servings of mashed potatoes with gravy (fat)

1 medium size steak or other deep fried meats (high animal protein and fat)
1 serving of chips and dips (salt and MSG)
Desserts: Ice cream or Super Cheese cake, Strawberry milk shake (sugar and fat)

After Dinner:
Potato chips or other kinds of processed chips and dips (salt, sugar, or MSG)
1 more cup of sugar soda because it tastes good with chips (sugar or Aspartame)

What's wrong with eating some or all of the above on a regular basis? Consider the following:

- High sugar will cause you to have mood swings and also put you on the highway to diabetes
- Caffeine will dehydrate you
- High animal protein is a possible cause of cancer in humans
- Oily food will let you experience weight increase, high blood pressure, high cholesterol, and possibly strokes or heart attacks!

4. How It's Supposed To Be

Junk food is supposed to be eaten for light entertainment only. As mentioned earlier, it should not be the main dish or a part of every meal.

If you choose not to be overweight or obese, then do not work against yourself by putting too much unhealthy food into your mouth. You are who you are today because of what and how you think and eat.

Recognize that junk food is great only for a few seconds per mouthful; it will be stuck in your body much longer until you work it out through hours of exercise or diet pills. Most of the junk food is turned into fat before it gets out, because if you have the habit of eating a lot of unhealthy food, before your stomach can work out the breakfast junk food, you are already heaping in a new batch of lunch junk! Before you know it, you will be adding another load of dinner junk to overwork your stomach and it goes on and on, day after day.

For example, All-You-Can-Eat Buffets are great and economical if you like to try different things and enjoy a variety of food for one price. The mistake many people make is that they think they *have* to eat all they can eat! They take it literally. Worst of all, they often plan out a strategy; for example, starving themselves and not eating or drinking anything until they hit the buffet. Or going for lots of the most expensive food items in the buffet, like steaks, BBQ spare ribs, and seafood, without considering the amount of salt, cholesterol, and fat that they will be adding to their poor bodies. How do I know so much? Been there, done that!

Do you dislike your body, or yourself, because you are overweight or obese? In case you do, it is time for you to renew your thoughts. Otherwise, it will only add more stress to your life. Recognize the following facts:

1. Your body shape and size is likely the result of genetics, how you think, and what you put into your mouth.
2. In order to stay healthy, besides genetics, it is your responsibility to eat less unhealthy food, avoid overeating, and guide your Inner thoughts (your Inner Voices – Chapter 7).

6
Jump Start With The "White Belt's Success Formula" – The Power of Water!

Before you read further, I would like to first introduce you to the Power of Water. The White Belt's Success Formula is the most basic strategy and it will help you get started. If you stick to the formula, you will soon realize that your cravings for soda or sugar drinks will be reduced, naturally. The following are the simple guidelines:

1. *Use formula for 6 days a week; take 1 day off from the formula per week.*
2. *Eat your breakfast, lunch, and dinner – no skipping. If you choose to spread out your breakfast, lunch, and dinner into 5 or 6 smaller meals, you are welcome to do so.*
3. *Avoid overeating.*
4. *Hungry between meals? Eat an organic apple, snack on carrot sticks, 100% whole grain crackers, organic cereals, or drink some water.*
5. *For best results: Walk around or on the spot for 10 – 15 minutes after each meal.*
6. *Finish your dinner at least 2.5 hours before bedtime – ideally, 3.5 hours ahead!*
7. *If you really have to have unhealthy snacks or soda, having them after your lunch is better than having junk food prior to sleeping.*
8. *Make it fun. Eat a variety of fresh fruits and vegetables every day!*

Let's Begin: Water type (Drink purified, distilled, or filtered water)

When you wake up

Drink 1 glass of water (8 oz = 1 Cup)

Breakfast:
½ - 1 glass of water
Your regular breakfast
½ - 1 glass of water

Between Meals: 1 glass of water

Lunch:
1 glass of water
Your regular lunch
1 glass of water

Between Meals: 1 glass of water

Dinner:
½ - 1 glass of water
Your regular dinner order
½ - 1 glass of water

1 glass of water two hours before you sleep

Sleep at least 8 hours per night whenever possible!

"Begin with the above White Belt's Success Formula now or starting tomorrow, if you like. By doing so, will speed up your journey to staying well! Have fun with it!"

7
Power Of Thought

How you think (Your Inner Voices: Inner Healthy Voice and Inner Junky Voice; plus, External Influence), will affect your eating, breathing, exercising, and resting habits, and this will eventually result in how you look and feel (Body – Health and Emotion). The cycle of unhealthy eating habits will go round and round if you do not take control over your thoughts.

MIND and BODY CHART (MAB Chart)

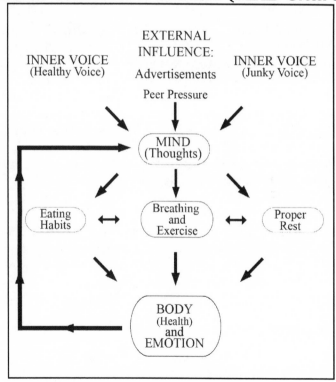

1) Get To Know Your Inner Twin (Inner Voices): Your "Inner Healthy Voice" and "Inner Junky (Junk Food) Voice"

Who are they?

Healthy Voice and Junky Voice are the two Inner Voices that each and every one of us is born with. They communicate with us throughout the day, discussing, negotiating, persuading, begging, requesting, and making demands of us either at the conscious or the subconscious level to eat or not to eat a certain food.

Your *Inner Healthy Voice* is the one that focuses on your *NEEDS (Eat To Live)*; usually it is your softer or ignored inner voice that tries to warn and stop you from overeating or eating too much junk food.

Your *Inner Junky Voice* is the one that focuses on your *WANTS (Live To Eat)*; your inner voice is very loud and bossy. It always begs, persuades, asks, forces, controls, demands, and drives you to overeat or eat all that junk food even though you know too much junk food is very harmful to you.

By getting to know both your Inner Voices job functions, you will have a good picture of how, why, and what could have been the causes of your being overweight or obese. With that understanding, this book will help you get back on track, one step at a time. Congratulations!

2) *Which Inner Voice Have You Been Listening To?*

Healthy Voice Or Junky Voice?

You will get a pretty good idea by looking into your current health condition or your appearance and your BMI. If you are currently suffering from health issues, such as high blood pressure, high cholesterol, other health challenges, or if you are overweight or obese, the answer is quite simple: You listen to your Inner Junky Voice more. And, you let it control you and dictate what you should eat; even when you know that unhealthy food is bad for you and even when you are full.

The difference between your needs (Inner Healthy Voice) and wants (Inner Junky Voice):

Needs are defined here as the healthy food you need to survive and stay healthy. Foods such as fresh fruits and vegetables, 100% whole grain, steamed and stir-fried foods are healthy.

Wants are defined here as junk food or food containing high sugar, salt, MSG, high animal protein, high oil or fat. For example, you do not *need* chocolate, cheesecake, potato chips, French-fries, steaks, or deep-fried chicken wings to survive.

If you listen to your Inner Junky Voice 80% of the time, it will fool around with you and eventually make your body hate you!!! Consciously or subconsciously, you will eat more and gain so much weight that you develop health problems. You will wake up in the morning and say, "Why is my body treating me like this?"

Your life will be transformed for the better, once you begin to take control over your Inner Junky Voice. Therefore, this book will guide you to eat right beginning with your power of thought.

By paying attention and listening to your Inner Healthy Voice, you will be informed of which kinds of food will bring immediate and long-term pain, and which kinds of food will bring wellness and long-term pleasure to your life.

How?

The next time you are craving junk food, simply quiet yourself down and you will start hearing suggestions coming into your mind like, "I'm so hungry now, I've got to eat something." Many times the chips and dips, burgers, fried food advertisements, or whatever unhealthy food advertisements that you watch the night before or those billboards or TV commercials will start flooding into your mind. If you are not paying attention to your thoughts, the advertisements will dictate what you should eat for the next meal.

However, if you choose to think before you eat and it happens that the only restaurant that is available to you is a junk food chain, you can still do something about it. For instance, the following is something you could do:

- Replace soda with water
- Order salad (limit your dressing to 2 tsp. of course) instead of fries
- Have a grilled lean meat sandwich instead of deep fried meat or a double cheeseburger

The choice is absolutely yours!

3) What To Do Now: Will Worry And Fear Help You Stay Healthy?

The answer is a big "NO." Instead of helping you and your body, worry and fear are often the culprits for bringing more stress into your life. Once you let worry, fear, and stress into your brain, your Inner Junky Voice will start talking, persuading, suggesting, asking, demanding, and compelling you to do things that will add more stress to your life. It might say something like, "Just eat those chips: they will calm me down," "Go for a large soda: it will bring my energy up," "How about ice cream? Yummy!!!" "Chocolate chips cookies, how can I resist," "All-I-Can-Eat Dinner Buffets..." Before you know it, you will have just loaded a ton of unhealthy foods into your stomach.

"We are grown ups with a kid inside everyone of us!" *That's why you still have to keep junk food out of your reach.* The easier you can reach it, the harder it will be for you to resist. Therefore, it is important to keep junk out of your house, whenever possible. Imagine this: it's midnight and you have a sudden urge to eat something, but there is no junk food in your house. You only have fresh fruits, organic cereal, oatmeal, and lightly salted organic crackers. What are you going to snack on in order to fulfill your urge? Answer: Fresh fruits, organic cereal, oatmeal, and lightly salted organic crackers.

However, if you stock up your junk food inventory at home as if a disaster is coming, the more likely you are to eat it and go out of control. How do I know so much about it? I have done that for years until my cholesterol reached 288 at the age of 25!

Accept the fact that you will be fine if you do not eat junk food at night even if your Inner Junky Voice calls for it. In fact, you will start to feel more in control the next morning if you managed to survive a night without eating junk. But, if it is too difficult for you to live without storing unhealthy food at home, you could do yourself the following favor:

- Avoid buying junk food in bulk
- Resist the buy-one-get-one-free junk food sale — the more you buy, the more you will eat
- Buy the smallest size available (save some money, save your health)
- Limit your junk food availability in your house whenever possible.

Always remember to give yourself a pat on the shoulder or say a "YES" with a fist pump for doing the right thing — resisting junk food temptations. Not only will you survive the night, you will not struggle as much to wake up in the morning. Instead, you will feel light-hearted and more energetic. In addition, you will feel great when you put on your clothes, because your stomach will not feel as bloated and your clothes should not feel as tight. Can you imagine what will happen to your looks, weight, and energy if you can resist the junk food temptations night after night?

Hint: Use the human inborn laziness — "procrastinate" to your advantage! Picture yourself having to change your clothes, drive, and waste your time and money just to buy junk food. If you crave it so much, and you actually go through all this trouble in the middle of the night, and you enjoy the junk food for a few minutes and then start to feel bad, you will learn from your mistake. And that is good, because this painful process will help you learn to procrastinate on your urge to eat unhealthy food next time! Just remember: MIND YOUR OWN WELLNESS is about changing habits. Once you have become good at procrastinating on eating junk food, you will learn to take control of your Inner Junky Voice when you are surrounded by junk food.

Positive Reminders: Always remind yourself that eating too much junk food is the major cause of your being overweight or obese, and it can only bring more pain to your life. If you link up junk food with pain and suffering frequently, you will soon train your mind to think of junk food as wants (Live To Eat), not needs (Eat To Live).

4) Beware Of Peer Pressure

How To Handle Them? Do not be affected by any of your peers' negative words!

Think for yourself, decide what's best for you and stick to it. Recognize the fact that your previous poor eating habits are the main reason that you are overweight.

Many people would want you to join them and eat food that tastes great, like deep fried foods, or treats high in sugar, salt, or trans fats. They'll feel better if you join them. So don't let your uninformed friends talk you into joining their unhealthy food feasts (unless it is your take-a-break day and you choose to do so). If your friends encourage you to eat junk food, just kindly reject it and stick to your game plan. Ultimately, you and only you are responsible to MIND YOUR OWN WELLNESS.

5) Let's Be Fair...

Be fair to yourself and be proud that you are taking up this challenge and are determined to shave off those unwanted pounds. If it took months or years for you to consistently follow the poor habit of eating to build those fat cells, it will take at least months to lose those extra pounds. Quick fixes are not the answer!

Accept this fact: Fat cannot be washed off like dirt on your hands.

Get ready: You already know how hard and costly it was to gain weight and maintain it. Now you have to choose to use that very same energy, but in the opposite direction!

It will be hard for you to fail with MIND YOUR OWN WELLNESS, because the 5 Color Belts' Success Formulas are *easy to follow.* By giving you the flexible choices from feeling OK with the White Belt's Success Formula to feeling great with the Black Belt's Success Formula, plus letting you know how to communicate with your Inner Twins (Healthy Voice and Junky Voice), there is little room for failure!

Be Patient and Persistent:

One essential step to success is to give yourself enough time and consistent encouragement for getting healthy.

Imagine yourself as a cruise ship. How do you turn it around? Answer: A single degree at a time. Likewise, if you take the time with your burning desire to pursue the staying healthy goal, you will make it, one pound at a time.

How? By making positive changes to:

1) Your eating habits
2) The way you feel and
3) How you control your Inner Junky Voice.

8
What Would Happen if...?

If you listen to your **Inner Junky Voice 80%** of the time, the following is usually what you get:

"Junky's Free Package":
- Overweight or obese
- Lowering of self esteem
- Shortness of breath
- Stiff neck
- High cholesterol
- High blood pressure
- Feeling tired most of the time
- Low energy
- Easily frustrated
- Moody
- Digestive problems
- Regular body ache
- Cancer
- Kidney diseases
- Heart diseases

If you do not pay attention to your inner voices and continue to eat 80% junk food and 20% healthy food, you can only expect your weight to continue to increase. And you know what that means!

However, if you pay attention to your **Inner Healthy Voice 80%** of the time, the following could happen to you:

- Save hundreds of dollars on junk foods per year
- Save hundreds to thousands of dollars on bigger sets of clothes, diet pills, liposuction surgery, etc...
- Increased self-esteem and confidence

- More energy and productivity
- Regularity without pills
- Fewer body aches
- Better sleep
- Feeling lighter
- Weight will go back to normal or at least closer to normal
- Normal breathing
- Lower cholesterol
- Minimized the chances of getting cancer, kidney, or heart diseases at a young age

Difference Between Healthy Voice And Junky Voice Food Choices

Junky Voice's Favorites:

- Deep fried food
- Especially shelled seafood – High in cholesterol
- Chocolate
- Chips
- Fries
- Steaks
- Pizza
- Soda
- High sugar juice or energy drink
- Coffee with sugar and whipped cream topping
- Buffets
- Dairy products (Chocolate milk, cheese, ice cream...)
- Candies
- White bread
- Cakes
- Ice-cold sugar drinks
- Desserts and other processed foods, etc...

Healthy Voice's Favorites:

- Minimize on all 14 Things (Chapter 2)
- Purified, distilled, or filtered water
- Wide variety of fresh fruits – preferably organic
- Fresh squeezed or blended fruit juice
- Fresh, steamed, or stir-fried vegetables – preferably dark green organics
- 100% whole grain, wheat with flax seed, whole wheat, or organic whole grain bread
- Oatmeal
- Oat bran
- Organic cereals
- Organic or whole wheat or grain pasta
- Less sugar — and use organic sugar whenever possible
- Less salt
- Replace enriched flour with organic or 100% whole grain flour
- Less meat – preferably lean meat over fatty meat
- Organic or 100% natural snacks
- Maximum 20% junk foods
- Live a healthier life

9
Beware Of Your Inner Junky Voice (IJV) - In 7 Situations...

Causes and Effects:

1. **Cause: "After you skip a meal..." – IJV yells!**
   Effect: You will eat too fast to satisfy your hunger, and you are likely to exceed your junk food limit before you recognize it.
   Solution: Drink a glass of water first, then deliberately slow down. Chew slower and chew your food well before you swallow it.

2. **Cause: "When you are very tired...it is hard to resist your Inner Junky Voice" – IJV shouts!**
   Effect: Overeating.
   Solution: Bring yourself to the present and remind yourself that adding junk food to your body or overeating could only make you feel more tired.
   a) Give yourself a 10 to 15 minute cat nap
   b) Drink a glass of water prior to eating
   c) Eat light - that will bring your energy back.

3. **Cause: "When you are stressed!" – IJV nags!**
   Effect: You will tend to eat junk food or overeat to get a sense of certainty.
   Solution: Recognize the fact that using junk food or overeating is not the way to reduce stress. Doing so will only relax you for the short time you are eating. Once you are done eating, you will have more stress in your life. Instead, go to a quiet place and close your eyes for a few minutes and take 10 deep breaths as follows:

"5-5-10 Exhale Breathing Exercise" (Chapter 12)
a) Breathe in for a silent count of 5 seconds
b) Hold your breath for the next 5 seconds
c) Exhale slowly for a count of 10.
d) Repeat a – c 10 times.

It's relaxing, free and it will not add pounds to your body.

4. **Cause: "When You Are Excited." – IJV cheers!**
   Effect: Eat more to slow down.
   Solution: Change your mental focus. Instead of listening to your Inner Junky Voice telling you to go for food, train yourself to switch your thoughts to doing something that will make you feel good, besides eating. Maybe you could write down your to-do list for the day or week, clean up your desk or room, go for a walk, read, exercise, or do the **"5-5-10 Exhale Breathing Exercise."**

5. **Cause: "Too hungry – waited too long till your next meal." – IJV screams!**
   Effect: "Your Wants" have been converted to "Your Needs," and your Inner Junky Voice will lead you to eat any food that is near you.
   Solution: This situation is similar to situation #1. Therefore, drink a glass of water, then deliberately slow down your eating speed by chewing slower and chewing your food well before you swallow it.

6. **Cause: "Lonely and Moody" – IJV cries!**
   Effect: Eat to kill time.
   Solution: Why not choose to do some volunteer work? Helping others = helping yourself to keep from over eating or eating too much unhealthy food. In addition, you may get to know someone who is nice to talk to or your special someone.

7. Cause: "*Extremely happy or Holiday seasons*" – IJV sings!

Effect: You are in the celebrating mood, wanting to overeat, too happy to worry about anything else.

Solution: This is a very strong emotion and it is very challenging to take full control, especially during holiday time. All kinds of sweets and salty temptations are floating around in your house and office...

For special holidays, it is okay to enjoy some treats. Just remind yourself to use at least the White Belt's Success Formula (Chapter 16) to guide you and AVOID OVEREATING. Instead of eating a huge slice of chocolate cake, just take a smaller slice. For instance, remind yourself that the more junk you put into your mouth this Christmas, the more of a bad start you will have for the coming New Year.

10
How To "Say NO" To Your Inner Junky Voice (IJV)!

You have probably noticed that junk foods often become more irresistible at night, during weekends, and on holidays. Why?

It has to do with trying to reward yourself for working hard during the day or week. It becomes very natural to give in to your Inner Junky Voice during these times. If you have just finished your dinner and your Inner Junky Voice is still trying to work on you, be firm and say "NO" (Self Talk), if you are determined to be healthy again.

How does your Inner Junky Voice work on you? Typically, it will start by flashing your favorite junk food into your mind – let's say, ice cream or chips and dips. Then it will start to nag you minute after minute until the junk food image reappears.

If you have never trained your Inner Healthy Voice to say "NO" to your favorite junk food, your Inner Junky Voice will gradually take control of your thoughts by creating vivid images of your favorite junk food until you convert the junk food from Want-To-Eat-It to a Need-To-Eat-It. Sometimes, your favorite junk food images could become so strong that you can almost smell or taste them through your imagination – this stage is called "You-Are-In-Trouble and Got-To-Eat-It!"

Sometimes the process could take minutes, and at other times you may just reach for your favorite junk without even thinking about it, because it is habit forming.

Here are some approaches to control your Inner Junky Voice.

1st Approach: The best way to say "NO" to your Inner Junky Voice is at the initial stage – when your favorite junk food first flashes into your mind. So, quiet down your mind and listen to your Inner Healthy Voice. It is trying to remind you that junk food is one of the main causes of your physical, mental, and financial pains.

2nd or Softer Approach: use your power of procrastination and say to your Inner Junky Voice, "I'll eat that tomorrow after lunch." Then stick to your decision. When tomorrow comes, there is a 50% chance that you might not feel like eating that junk food at all. So, don't force it down your throat, just because you said you could.

In order to use this approach, it is crucial for you to keep your favorite junk foods out of reach, whenever possible. The harder or the more inconvenient it is for you to get or purchase your junk food, the better the chances of your success. Otherwise, you will have to put yourself through a tough test of resisting and not eating your favorite junk food that is right before your face.

3rd or Toughest Approach: When your favorite junk food is in front of you and it is late at night and you are hungry. What should you do?

i.   First drink a glass of water.
ii. Decide that you desire better health over junk food.
iii. Remind yourself that your favorite junk food is one of the main culprits of your current pains and you do not need it now.
iv. Put it away or throw it out.
v.   Give yourself a pat on your back or make a fist and say "YES" for resisting the temptation.
vi. If, your hunger does not go away, eat a slice or two of organic or 100% whole grain bread (or toast it) with a teaspoon of 100% pure honey or raw almond butter, or have a small bowl of oatmeal (avoid instant oatmeal that comes with coloring, preservatives, artificial flavoring, and sugar).

vii. Next time around, make your life simpler, keep junk food out of your reach and go to bed earlier, whenever possible, so that you will not have to eat before bedtime.

11
Watch Out For "Advertisements" And Your Inner Junky Voice:

How do food advertisements shape our lives? By seduction!

First, the advertisement gets in front of your eyes in many ways:

- Television advertisements – you are bombarded with seductive, mouth-watering images.
- Newspapers or magazines' advertisements – for those who do not watch TV
- Direct mailings – advertisements that get in your mailbox, in case you do not watch TV and do not read newspapers or magazines
- Billboard advertisements – huge advertisements that are placed along the highways, in case you do not watch TV, do not read newspapers or magazines, and do not open your mailbox.
- Door-To-Door advertisements – advertisements that is hung on your door knob, in case you do not drive, you do not watch TV, do not read newspapers or magazines, and do not open the mailbox.
- Internet advertisements – in case you do not do any of the above activities, but do go online.

Actually, the point of advertising is not just to reach you once. The goal is to hit you over the head as many times as possible. That is the reason you will often see the same advertiser advertising on all the different channels. The more ways and the more times that their advertisements can appear in front of your face, the better chance they will have to shape your decisions and habits in order to motivate you to purchase their foods or things.

Adults are not the only ones who are being bombarded by advertisers. Children too are being targeted, especially if their main source of entertainment is TV. In fact, children are even more vulnerable than adults to advertisements because of their innocence. If you are not aware of what the food advertisers are doing to your kids, you may end up being influenced and persuaded by your children to buy what they want and like to eat – as seen on TV, whether it is good or bad for their health.

If you are unaware of what and how food advertisers are doing to your brain, it will soon create cravings in you and train your Inner Junky Voice to talk to you in the following ways:

- "It's Holiday Season - Oh my...those expensive chocolate gifts in the office... I would never make or buy if I had to pay for it myself...it is now free...I better eat all I can or I might miss out!"
- "Goodness...those chocolate drops will melt in my mouth!"
- "Creamy desserts...Yum!"
- "BBQ ribs...tender, juicy...got to have them!"
- "¼ pound juicy BBQ steaks!"
- "See that set of three delicious chocolates, why not just try one, then just one more, after that, why not finish it all?" "Oooooh... those chocolate dipped strawberries!"
- "Yum...Yum...those irresistible rippled chips and dips!"
- "Free ice cream samples... Why not?"
- "Super Buffet...I am going to eat whatever I can – fries, cheesecakes, pies, cookies, ice-cream, shrimp, sausages, fried wings, steaks...after all, I have already paid for it!"
- "All-I-Can-Eat bacon, ham and cheese breakfast, Eat All-I-Want spare ribs lunch, Eat-Till-I-Drop Blood clogging, cholesterol building Deep-Fried Seafood Buffet Dinner!

Awareness:

Recognize the fact that you are born with your Inner Twins (Healthy Voice and Junky Voice) and realize that your Inner Junky Voice often gets the upper hand if you are facing the challenge of overweight or obesity. Once you learn to say "NO!" to your Inner Junky Voice, your Inner Healthy Voice will return to take good care of your body.

In addition, if you have children, once you learn the ways to MIND YOUR OWN WELLNESS, you will be able to give your children a gift that will last for the rest of their lives.

12
Breathing and Physical Exercise — What do they have to do with Staying Healthy?

Besides keeping you alive, do you know that oxygen is the gas that gives your body natural energy? What about carbon dioxide? It is not just the gas that you breathe out; it is a harmful waste gas that you are supposed to get rid of.

If you desire better health, it is important to constantly remind yourself to take deep breaths. Although taking deep breaths may sound like a no-brainer, deep breathing exercises are often neglected when you are caught in a stressful situation. When you are worried or stressed, you will have a tendency to take shorter breaths because your heart is pumping so quickly and things get out of control for you.

If you are not aware that taking a deep breath can calm you and slow down your breathing, your Inner Junky Voice will jump right in and tell you to reach for junk food to slow you down whether you are hungry or not, just to regain control.

If you train yourself to take a deep breath regularly, your natural energy level will increase and you will be able to handle stress well instead of using junk food to cope with stress.

Bottom Line: Inhale the natural energy in oxygen and exhale the toxic waste from carbon dioxide to help you deal with stress. It's free and it will not increase your weight.

By using junk food to manage stress, you will get stressed. Once you are done with the junk food, your stress level will actually go up because you have just wasted your money on junk food and added more fat or weight to your body.

Fun breathing exercise #1:

"Breathe like a PRO! Breathe like a BABY – Through Your Diaphragm!"

1. Sit down on a comfortable chair
2. Put both feet on the ground and straighten your back (for best results)
3. Lower your chin a little, so that you can see your stomach
4. Simply place your LEFT hand on your CHEST and RIGHT hand on your STOMACH.
5. Exhale slowly with your lips almost shut and make the "SSS..." sound as long as you can (Without feeling uncomfortable or out of breath)
6. Then inhale fully and see which hand rises
7. If your RIGHT hand rises more than your LEFT hand, you are mostly breathing through your diaphragm – Good for you!
8. But, if your LEFT hand or chest rises more than your RIGHT hand, you are mostly breathing through your lungs and not your diaphragm; which is not as good for you because breaths taken in through lungs only, are usually short and shallow. In other words, you are not giving your body as much oxygen as it needs. Once your breaths become shorter and shorter, you are likely to experience a headache, become tired, or stressed.

How do you learn to breathe through your diaphragm? Practice! Repeat steps 1 – 6 until you start seeing your RIGHT hand rising and your stomach expanding. You will get it soon. Both you and I were born with this talent, however once our lungs were fully developed, we started to breathe mostly through our lungs instead of our diaphragms. All we need to do is relearn the proper breathing technique.

Remind yourself regularly to breathe through your diaphragm until it becomes your second nature, especially when you are caught in stressful situations.

Another fun and relaxing breathing exercise:

"5-5-10 Exhale"

Do the following breathing exercise 3 or more times a day:

1. **Inhale for a count of 5**
2. **Hold for the next count of 5**
3. **Exhale slowly for a count of 10**
4. **Repeat 1. – 3. for 10 times.**

Benefits of this exercise:

- Keeps you calm and relaxed
- Increases your energy level
- Eases tension
- Relieves stress so as to prevent you from using junk food to slow you down
- Helps you stay focused on your goals

Physical Exercises

When you exercise, your heart will beat faster and you will breathe deeper. Doing so will help you squeeze carbon dioxide (toxic gas) out of your body and replenish it with FAT FREE oxygen to energize you naturally. By exercising regularly (walking, golfing, jogging, stretching, swimming, Yoga, Tai-chi, cardio workout, or other forms of physical exercise), you will get these benefits:

1. Deep breathing (mentioned earlier) or breathing through diaphragm (watch how a newborn baby does it: stomach bloats when inhaling, stomach collapses when exhaling).
2. More energy during the day – due to deep breathing.
3. Less urge to eat junk food.
4. Sleep better at night.
5. Reduce stress due to better rest.
6. Better concentration due to better sleep.
7. Burn more fat than just by sitting.
8. Boost your immune system with good blood circulation.
9. Feel great physically, mentally, and emotionally.

Exercise

"Along with a healthy diet, exercise is important for cancer prevention and survival. Exercise helps trim excess weight and may strengthen the immune defenses. Establishing a regular exercise program, along with a healthy diet, is extremely beneficial for everyone and is ever important in tackling cancer."[30]

13
Sleep — What does it have to do with staying healthy?

Sleep To Stay Energized:

Notice that children always seem restless? Do you realize that children are almost always doing a couple more things than adults do?

- They run around (exercise) more than we do and
- They almost always sleep 1 to 4 hours more a night than we do.

By exercising more, they get better and deeper sleep through diaphragm breathing. And by sleeping more hours than we do, they seem to have much more energy than adults.

As adults, we often convince ourselves that after a hard day of work, we need to have a good hour of television to relax our brain. But that one hour is likely to turn into 3 to 5 hours of a brain stressing TV-watching workout, because around the 5th hour, we've only left ourselves time for 4 to 6 hours of sleep before we have to get up in the morning. No wonder we are often more tired than kids.

For example:

If you sleep only five hours a day and convert one hour of TV watching time to sleep, you could increase your sleep by 20%. By cutting back two hours of TV time to sleep, you could increase your sleep time by 40%. What a deal!

What do you think would happen to your ability to cope with stress, your productivity, your health, etc?

As sleep expert Dr. James B. Maas of Cornell University stated in his book: *Power Sleep*, *"The process of sleep, if given adequate time and the proper environment...restores, rejuvenates, and energizes the body and brain. A third of your life spend sleeping has profound effects on the other two thirds of your life, in terms of alertness, energy, mood, body weight, perception, memory, thinking, reaction time, productivity, performance, communication skills, creativity, safety, and good health."*[31]

To some, sleeping more than five hours a day is a waste of time. I used to think that way too!

But think about the number of times that you dozed off during the day while working and worst of all, what if you dozed off while driving when alertness and safety become the big factors. Whether it is on-the-job safety or traffic safety, it is important for all of us to sleep at least 8 hours per night whenever possible.

Side effects of lack of sleep:

- Decreased productivity
- Need caffeine or sugar to wake up
- Side effects from caffeine and sugar complicate things
- Dizziness
- Heart pumps much faster than normal
- Shortness of breath
- Fatigue
- Nausea
- Get sick often due to improper rest
- Increase the chances of fatal accidents

The following are some important facts. According to:

- National Sleep Foundation's 2005 Sleep in America poll: "60% of adult drivers – about 168 million people – say they have driven a vehicle while feeling drowsy in the past year, and more than one-third, (37% or 103 million people), have actually fallen asleep at the wheel! In fact, of those who have nodded off, 13% say they have done so at least once a month. Four percent – approximately 11 million drivers – have had an accident or near accident because they dozed off or were too tired to drive."[32]

- National Highway Traffic Safety Administration (US): at least "100,000 police-reported crashes are direct result of driver fatigue each year. The results is an estimated 1,550 deaths, 71,000 injuries, and $12.5 billion in monetary lost."[33]

- Wall Street Journal: "$70 billion is lost per year in productivity, accidents, and health costs as a result of workers' inability to adjust to late-night work schedules."[34]

According to Gallup surveys, *"56% of the adult population now reports daytime drowsiness as a problem. The cost of sleep deprivation is nothing short of devastating in terms of wasted education and training, impaired performance, diminished productivity, loss of income, accidents, illness, the quality of life, and loss of life."*[35]

Don't be a victim and don't victimize innocent drivers, passengers, pedestrians, and others who happen to be near you just because you are lacking sleep. Sleep at least 8 hours everyday, whenever possible. Missing some late-night TV programs and advertisements is far better than sitting in a court trying to explain away your guilt in front of a judge and jury. Television programs can be very relaxing, as long as you are not sacrificing your precious sleeping hours for it. Even better, record your favorite late-night programs and watch them during your day off. Think counter clockwise: If you have to wake up at 7am, your sleeping time is 11pm or earlier; if you have to be up by 6am, it is best to sleep by 10pm, etc...

14
One Action
Can Change Your Life...
Physically, Mentally, and
Financially

Put less unhealthy food into your mouth (sugar, MSG, saturated fat, trans fat...) **VERSUS** dealing the with following challenges:

Physically:
- Headache
- Dizziness
- Feeling like vomiting or throwing up
- Stomach discomfort
- Acne problem
- Tired and sleepy
- Stiff neck or neck pain
- Losing concentration or focus
- Dozing off during meeting or work
- Overweight
- Gaining more and more weight
- Constipation
- Shortness of breath
- Face and body keep expanding
- Decrease in energy
- Slowing down or less productive due to overweight
- Reduction in productivity – could lead to job problems
- Speeding up heart diseases and other serious health problems

Mentally:
- Stress
- Mood swings

- Lower self-esteem
- Lower self-confidence
- Feeling hopeless
- Feeling stress
- Disliking yourself more and more everyday
- Losing control and eat more and more junk food
- Quit looking at yourself in the mirror all together, etc...
- Decreased motivation
- Worrying about diseases

Financially:
- Wasting hundreds of dollars on diet programs with yoyo effects
- Spending hundreds to thousands of dollars for bigger sized clothes
- Wasting more money on junk food
- Spending money on dieting pills
- Spending thousands of dollars on liposuction surgeries

Affecting Others:
- Becoming less patient with people who are around you
- Worrying your loved ones due to your poor health conditions

Gone Forever: Leaving your loved ones and friends prematurely forever, because of poor eating habits.

Health Is Like Wealth!

If you do not take care of your body, it is like you are not taking care of your money. Eat it all and you will waste it all. Notice that most of us are lucky to be born healthy. One of the main reasons that people become overweight or obese at a young age and face health challenges, such as high blood pressure, high cholesterol, diabetes, and heart disease, is overeating unhealthy food.

If you limit the portion of junk food that you eat and combine it with high fiber and healthier food such as fresh fruits and vegetables (but not from cans – canned foods are usually very high in salt and/or sugar), you are likely going to prolong your life for future enjoyment of all kinds of food. Eat *what* you want, not all you want! Minimize the junk!

Staying healthy has to do with "What and How" you eat!

Some of us exercise to lose weight; but some exercise to eat more. Not that we want to eat more, but our Inner Junky Voice tells us that by exercising more, it is OK to eat more and not gain weight (the same as exercising to loose two pounds so that you can eat more because now you have two pounds worth of room for junk food).

Think before you eat unhealthy food! Without a doubt, it is easy to get the entire big bag of delicious chips, a pint of ice cream, or a bag of cookies into your stomach within a short period of time. Please note:

1. You are what you eat!

2. Overeating will not sit well with your stomach. You don't want to medicate your eating habits or to medicate your medicine habits.

3. Your money could be drained away for medical bills because of your poor eating habits.

4. Worst of all, it will put you on a highway to major health challenges.

Special Attention:

It is normal for kids to have some treats and surprises from time to time. Likewise, your Inner Twins – Inner Healthy Voice and Inner Junky Voice are like real kids too.

If you are deprived of surprises (absolutely no junk food at all for too long – weeks or months), your Inner Healthy Voice may quit on you and stop giving advice to you on what not to eat - thereby causing the yoyo diet effect again.

From time to time, you will need to give yourself a break and that is where the 20% of your Inner Junky Voice comes into play. By being flexible and capping off your junk food intake to 20% per meal, per day, or per week, you will have the key to this MIND your own WELLNESS program. Be flexible and be firm with your Inner Junky Voice when you need to.

As always, pay attention to your Inner Voices and recognize which one is talking to you. Take control of your thoughts!

Just remember, your Inner Junky Voice will always try to influence you to eat more junk food than you need and your Inner Healthy Voice will continue to do its best to cap off your junk to 20% maximum.

Key to the solutions:

Reverse your 80% junk food and 20% healthy food eating habits to 80% or more healthy food and 20% or less junk food and you will see positive changes to your body, weight, and health!

15
Your 3 Choices To Better Health

All the Color Belts' Success Formulas apply to only six days a week. You will always get a one day break per week. And during your take-a-break day, you can choose to continue to eat light or you can eat as you did before you learned about MIND YOUR OWN WELLNESS.

Observation and Awareness: During your take-a-break-day, make mental notes of what you eat and how it affects your energy, stress level, mood, breathing, how you feel — heavy or light, comfortable or uncomfortable, happy or sad — after you eat and also how you feel the next morning. What you eat the night before will affect you the next day.

For example, if you eat heavily or overeat the night before, the junk food in your stomach will mess up your breathing and sleeping patterns, which will directly impact your energy level and your mood the next day. Always remember the pain and discomfort that overeating, or eating too much junk food, brings you.

Ask your Inner Healthy Voice to remind you of the pains you have gotten from overeating or over-dosing yourself with the particular group of unhealthy foods. This will help you break away from bad eating habits and replace them with good ones sooner. The sooner you manage to associate those bad experiences with overeating and unhealthy food, the sooner you can break free. The choice is absolutely yours.

If you choose to eat only heavy meals during lunch (and eat light during dinner) on your take-a-break day, your energy level should go down only during the day and you should feel better the next morning as compared to eating junk for the whole day during your take-a-break day. Have fun with the process and do not cheat. Once you take control of your thinking, you'll realize that the whole wide world isn't going to collapse just because you don't get to eat junk food and you can laugh at the junk food and tell it you are too smart to take it seriously anymore!

Method #1:

First, decide when you would like to have your take-a-break day and stick to it as long as your schedule allows. Be flexible when you need to.

For example, if you pick every Thursday (middle of the week) to be your take-a-break day:

Week #1: White Belt Strategy (Mon-Wed; Thu (take-a-break); Fri-Sun)
Week #2: Green Belt Strategy (Mon-Wed; Thu (take-a-break); Fri-Sun)
Week #3: Purple Belt Strategy (Mon-Wed; Thu (take-a-break); Fri-Sun)
Week #4: Red Belt Strategy (Mon-Wed; Thu (take-a-break); Fri-Sun)
Week #5: Black Belt Strategy (Mon-Wed; Thu (take-a-break); Fri-Sun)

- As always, sleep at least 8 hours per night whenever you can.
- Record your favorite late-night TV programs, shut your TV off, and go to bed.

The reason that the White Belt's Success Formula is used for week #1 and then Green Belt's Success Formula for the next and so on, is because we, as humans, are creatures of habit. A sudden change with what we used to eat could create uneasiness.

Be flexible and do not beat yourself up if you are not able to stick with the darker color belts due to the change in your eating patterns. Just remember one thing, hydrate yourself with water, not soda or coffee, and stick to at least the White Belt's Success Formula. If you are really craving soda or coffee, drink it after you drink 1 – 2 portions of water. Fair enough?

Once you are through with the Black Belt's Success Formula and feeling the positive effects that the Color Belt's Success Formulas bring you physically and mentally, you can pick and choose whichever color belt you like to stick with or switch it around as needed. Do your best to stick with the darker color belts (Purple and up).

What about party time, birthdays, holidays? Stick to at least the White Belt's Success Formula.

Method #2:

Likewise, decide when you would like to have your take-a-break day and stick with it as long as your schedule allows. Be flexible when you have to.

If you are currently overweight (BMI between 25 and 29) or in the obese stage (BMI = 30 and over), you could jump right into the Red or Black Belt's Success Formula, as long as you choose to manage the positive change with your eating habits.

The longer you can stick to and get used to good eating habits (Purple, Red, or Black Belt's Formula), the sooner you can get healthier, naturally. Give yourself the power and authority to take full control of your thoughts and you will be pleasantly surprised with the way you look, the way you think and feel in the weeks, months, and years to come. You can do it! Go for it!

Method #3:

You could pick and choose different color belts for breakfast, lunch, and dinner. However, this method will not be the best for you if you are always telling yourself that you are so busy that all you can do is to stay on the White or Green Belt's Success

Formula only. Move up to the darker color belts – help yourself to get healthy and start focusing on the looks and good health that you desire! Get it with MIND YOUR OWN WELLNESS! Like Napoleon Hill said, "Be Patient, Be Persistent!"

16
5 Color Belts' Success Formulas — How Do They Work?

Taking Charge: 5 Color Belts To Help You...*What color is your belt today?* Take one day off from the Formula per week!

	(Healthy Food / Junky Food)	Success	
White Belt	*(10% / 90%)*	Level	1
Green Belt	*(20% / 80%)*	Level	2
Purple Belt	*(40% / 60%)*	Level	3
Red Belt	*(60% / 40%)*	Level	4
Black Belt	*(80% / 20%)*	Level	5

A) Weigh yourself 1st thing in the morning = _____ pounds

B) Find out what your weight would be if your BMI is at 24. Refer to the BMI (Body Mass Index) chart in Chapter 5 (page 89). What would your normal weight be: _____ pounds, if your BMI is at 24.

C) Take your weight on (A) minus (B)

For example: If you are 6' (foot) tall—
        A) Your current weight = 206 pounds
        B) BMI at 24 = 177 pounds
Take (A) − (B) = 206 − 177 = 29 extra pounds of opportunities to let go.

Common Difference Between Black Belt Success Formula and Take A Break Day

Black Belt's Formula	Versus	Take-A-Break Day (Junk Food Day)

Feel Light
Not Bloated
Feel Healthy
Energetic

Feel Heavy
Feel Bloated
Feel Sick
Lack Energy

What Color Is Your Belt?

You do not need to start from White Belt, if you are already drinking enough water. You could give yourself a pat on the back and begin with Green Belt and enjoy your way up to the Black Belt's Success Formula.

Week #1: White Belt's Success Formula: For
total Junkies, just like me for 20 years, and also a good start for Heavy Soda or Coffee Users —

The purpose of the White Belt's Success Formula is to let you get used to drinking enough water without changing your routine eating habit.

- And you may ask, "If I drink so much water, where do I find room for my soda and junk food?"
- Answer: That's the main purpose of this book – reducing your craving for sugar drinks and junk foods by filling your body with water and healthier foods – Without going hungry!

Week #2: Green Belt: Good belt to start for anyone
who drinks at least 8 glasses of water a day; but, hardly experiences the benefits of eating fresh fruits and vegetables.

Week #3: Purple Belt: Great belt to begin for anyone who drinks enough water and eats only a small portion of fresh fruits and vegetables a day.

Week #4 and #5: Red and Black Belts: Get your health and weight back on track and stay on track.

Red and Black Belts' Success Formulas will help you bring your weight and BMI back (or at the very least) close to normal and let you enjoy the priceless benefits of staying healthy!

- Increase energy and productivity
- Increase self-esteem and confidence
- Love yourself more than ever
- Reduce your chance of getting health diseases at a young age

Be flexible! You can switch around the 5 Color Belts' Success Formulas throughout the day depending on your situation. Just use the same rule of thumb – if you choose to have better health, use Red or Black Formula 4 to 5 days a week and make it your routine. Just remember, when you are invited for a party, use at least the White Belt's Success Formula – drink one to two portions of water first then start eating and avoid overeating. Have fun with it.

Please Note:
1 Portion = the size of your fist; ½ portion = about ½ the size of your fist
1 Glass of water = 8 oz or 1 cup
Water Choices:
- **Drink purified, distilled, or filtered water**

Alex Ong

"For total junk food junkies – just like me for 20 years!"

White Belt's Success Formula: 10/90

White Belt:

- When you drink a glass of water before you eat, it will reduce your craving for soda or coffee, naturally; because your body's need for fluid has been fulfilled by water, instead of sugar drinks.
- Your desire for more salty food will also be reduced because water tends to neutralize your taste buds rather than activate your cravings for salty food.
- If you have added 1 to 2 glasses of water to every one of your regular meals without overeating, you have just reduced your white sugar and junk food intake by 10 to 20 percent, naturally. Because water does take up space in your stomach.

Results of using the White Belt's Success Formula:

Your will feel a little lighter, happier, and more energetic consistently throughout the day.

Green Belt's Success Formula: 20/80

Green Belt = (White Belt's positive effects + one portion of fresh fruits or vegetables)

- By adding 1 to 2 glasses of water and 1 portion of fresh fruits or vegetables to every one of your regular meals, you are adding natural fiber and antioxidants to your body.
- Besides reducing your sugar and unhealthy food intake, you will have more regular digestive habits because of the natural fiber from fresh fruits or vegetables that you ate.
- In addition, the antioxidants that you get from the fresh fruits and vegetables will strengthen your immune system and make you healthier or look younger.
- If you drink (add) one to 2 glasses of water and one portion of fresh fruits or vegetables to all of your regular meals without overeating, you have just reduced your regular sugar and junk food intake by 20 to 30 percent, naturally.

Results of using the Green Belt's Success Formula:

- Feel lighter + happier
- More energetic throughout the day
- Better digestion
- Get sick less
- Younger looking

Purple Belt's Success Formula: 40/60

Purple Belt = (Green Belt's positive effects + ½ to 1 more portion of fresh fruits or vegetables)

- By adding 1 to 2 glasses of water and 1½ to 2 portions of fresh fruits or vegetables to all of your regular meals, you are adding 1.5 to 2 times as much natural fiber and antioxidants to your body.
- Besides reducing your sugar and junk food intake, you will have better digestive habits because of the natural fiber from fresh fruits or vegetables that you eat.
- Like the Green Belt's routine, the antioxidants that you get from the fruits and vegetables will strengthen your immune system and make you healthier and look younger.
- If you drink 1 to 2 glasses of water and add 1½ to 2 portions of fresh fruits or vegetables to every one of your regular meals and avoid overeating, you have just reduced your regular sugar and junk food intake by 40 to 50 percent, naturally!

Results of using the Purple Belt's Success Formula:

- Feel lighter
- More energetic throughout the day
- Better digestion
- Get sick less
- Younger looking
- Better concentration or more productive at work
- Better sleep

Red Belt's Success Formula: 60/40

Red Belt = (Purple Belt's positive effects + eating light and healthy for breakfast and dinner)

- By adding 1 to 2 glasses of water and 2 to 3 portions of fresh fruits or vegetables to all of your regular meals and eating light and healthy for breakfast and dinner, you are not only adding twice as much natural fiber and antioxidants to your body, you are taking burdens away from your body in the morning and at night.
- Eating light for breakfast will give you a good energetic start for the day and eating light for dinner will help you sleep better. In addition, you are less likely to struggle to wake up in the next morning because your stomach, kidneys, and liver will not have to work as hard while you sleep during the night.
- Like the Purple Belt's routine, the antioxidants that you get from the fruits, vegetables and, lighter and healthier meals will enhance your immune system, help you look younger, and energize you without the help of caffeine, energy drinks, or diet pills.
- If you drink 1 to 2 glasses of water and 2 to 3 portions of fresh fruits or vegetables to all of your regular meals and eat light and healthy in the morning and at night (without overeating), you have just reduced your regular sugar and junk food intake by 60 to 70 percent, naturally.
- Your excess weight will start to go down. The heavier you are now, the bigger the change you will notice when you follow the Red Belt's Success Formula.

Results of using the Red Belt's Success Formula:

- Feel lighter and start to weigh less
- More energetic throughout the day
- Better digestion
- Get sick less
- Younger looking
- Better concentration or more productive at work
- Better sleep
- Notice the drop in weight
- Your clothes will start to loosen up
- Some body aches and pains may also go away, naturally

Black Belt's Success Formula: 80/20

Black Belt = (Red Belt's positive effects + eating light and healthy 6 days a week)

- Eating light and healthy for 6 days a week is the best formula for a healthy life. If you can eat light and healthy for 7 days a week, that is even better, however that is harder to achieve for most people, including myself!
- The main reason that MIND YOUR OWN WELLNESS works is because of the following:
  o It allows you to be flexible with what to eat, in case you have a sudden change of plans or schedules.
  o You are given the control over how fast you want to loose that excess weight.
  o Your Color Belts' Success Formulas are your road-block to the yoyo diet effect because you are not forced to stop eating your favorite junk food. All you need to do is to minimize it. Plus, you always have one day a week to eat what or all you want (just remember to note how you feel after eating too much unhealthy food or eating all you want).
  o It educates you as to how unhealthy food and overeating habits affect your health.
  o It gives you the facts and reasons as to why it is important to minimize eating the 14 Common Things (Chapter 2) that can be in your food and it shows you how to replace your unhealthy food with healthy food, naturally; through the 5 Color Belts' Success Formulas.
  o The formulas are direct and easy to follow.
  o It shows you the way to use the Power of Your Thought to help you get on track and stay on track.

Results of using the Black Belt Formula:

- Feel lighter and start to weigh less
- More energetic throughout the day
- Better digestion
- Get sick less
- Younger looking
- Better concentration

- Better sleep
- Notice the drop in weight
- Your clothes will start to loosen up
- You can give your "big sized" clothes to charities
- Most of your body aches and pains may go away, naturally
- Some of your allergies may disappear
- Increase the chance of reversing chronic illnesses or diseases
- Live your healthiest and best!

Apply the following 8 points to all 5 Color Belts' Success Formulas:

1. *Use formula for 6 days a week; take 1 day off from the formula per week.*
2. *Eat your breakfast, lunch, and dinner – no skipping. If you choose to spread out your breakfast, lunch, and dinner into 5 or 6 smaller meals, you are welcome to do so.*
3. *Avoid overeating.*
4. *Hungry between meals? Eat an organic apple, snack on carrot sticks, 100% whole grain crackers, organic cereals, or drink some water.*
5. *For best results: Walk around or on the spot for 10 – 15 minutes after each meal.*
6. *Finish your dinner at least 2.5 hours before bedtime – ideally, 3.5 hours ahead!*
7. *If you really have to have unhealthy snacks or soda, having them after your lunch is better than having junk food prior to sleeping.*
8. *Make it fun. Eat a variety of fresh fruits and vegetables every day!*

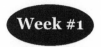

White Belt's Success Formula: 10/90

1 glass of water once you are awake

Breakfast:
½ to 1 glass of water
Your regular breakfast order
½ to 1 glass of water

Between Meals: 1 glass of water

Lunch:
1 glass of water
Your regular lunch order
1 glass of water

Between Meals: 1 glass of water

Dinner:
½ to 1 glass of water
Your regular dinner order
½ to1 glass of water

1 glass of water 2 hours before you sleep

Sleep at least 8 hours per night whenever possible!

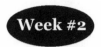
Week #2

Green Belt's Success Formula: 20/80

1 glass of water once you are awake

Breakfast:
½ to 1 glass of water
1 portion of fresh fruits or vegetables (eat fresh, blend, juice, or squeeze)
Your regular breakfast order
½ to 1 glass of water

Between Meals: 1 glass of water

Lunch:
1 glass of water
1 portion of fresh fruits or vegetables (eat fresh, blend, juice, or squeeze)
Your regular lunch order
1 glass of water

Between Meals: 1 glass of water

Dinner:
½ to 1 glass of water
1 portion of fresh, steamed, or stir-fried green leaf vegetables
Your regular dinner order
½ to 1 glass of water

1 glass of water 2 hours before you sleep

Sleep at least 8 hours per night whenever possible!

Week #3

Purple Belt's Success Formula: 40/60

1 glass of water once you are awake

Breakfast:
½ to 1 glass of water
1.5 to 2 portions of fresh fruits or vegetables (eat fresh, blend, juice, or squeeze)
Your regular breakfast order
½ to 1 glass of water

Between Meals: 1 glass of water

Lunch:
1 glass of water
1.5 to 2 portions of fresh fruits or vegetables (eat fresh, steamed, or stir-fried green leaf vegetables)
Your regular lunch order
1 glass of water

Between Meals: 1 glass of water

Dinner:
½ to 1 glass of water
1.5 to 2 portions of fresh fruits or vegetables (eat fresh, steamed, or stir-fried green leaf vegetables)
Your regular dinner order
½ to 1 glass of water

1 glass of water 2 hours before you sleep

Sleep at least 8 hours per night whenever possible!

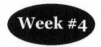

Red Belt's Success Formula: 60/40

1 glass of water once you are awake

Breakfast:
½ to 1 glass of water
2 to 3 portions of fresh fruits or vegetables (eat fresh or Juice)
2 portions of 100% whole grain sandwich, whole grain cereal with almond milk, or oatmeal
½ to 1 glass of water

Between Meals: 1 glass of water

Lunch:
1 glass of water
2 to 3 portions of fresh fruits or vegetables (eat fresh, steamed, or stir-fried green leaf vegetables)
Your regular lunch order
1 glass of water

Between Meals: 1 glass of water

Dinner:
½ to 1 glass of water
2 to 3 portions of fresh fruits or stir-fried green leaf vegetables
2 portions of 100% whole grain food (pasta, bread, or rice) or beans
½ portion of stir-fried, baked, or steamed (fish or lean meat) dish, if needed
½ to 1 glass of water

1 glass of water 2 hours before you sleep

Sleep at least 8 hours per night whenever possible!

Black Belt's Success Formula: 80/20

1 glass of water once you are awake

Breakfast:
½ to 1 glass of water
2 to 3 portions of fresh fruits or vegetables (eat fresh, blend, juice, or squeeze)
2 portions of 100% whole grain sandwich, whole grain cereal with almond milk, or oatmeal
½ to 1 glass of water

Between Meals: 1 glass of water

Lunch:
1 glass of water
2 to 3 portions of fresh fruits or vegetables (eat fresh, steamed, or stir-fried green leaf vegetables)
2 portions of 100% whole grain food (pasta, bread, or rice) or beans
½ portion of grilled (fish or lean meat) dish, if needed
1 glass of water

Between Meals: 1 glass of water

Dinner:
½ to 1 glass of water
2 to 3 portions of fresh fruits or vegetables (eat fresh, steamed, or stir-fried green leaf vegetables)
2 portions of 100% whole grain food (pasta, bread, or rice) or beans
½ portion of stir-fried, baked, steamed, or grilled (fish or lean meat) dish, if needed
½ to 1 glass of water

1 glass of water 2 hours before you sleep

Sleep at least 8 hours per night whenever possible!

Sample Menus:
Green Belt *To* Black Belt

"Just A Reminder"

Apply the following 8 points to all 5 Color Belts' Success Formulas:

1. *Use formula for 6 days a week; take 1 day off from the formula per week.*
2. *Eat your breakfast, lunch, and dinner – no skipping. If you choose to spread out your breakfast, lunch, and dinner into 5 or 6 smaller meals, you are welcome to do so.*
3. *Avoid overeating.*
4. *Hungry between meals? Eat an organic apple, snack on carrot sticks, 100% whole grain crackers, organic cereals, or drink some water.*
5. *For best results: Walk around or on the spot for 10 – 15 minutes after each meal.*
6. *Finish your dinner at least 2.5 hours before bedtime – ideally, 3.5 hours ahead!*
7. *If you really have to have unhealthy snacks or soda, having them after your lunch is better than having junk food prior to sleeping.*
8. *Make it fun. Eat a variety of fruits and vegetables every day!*

Green Belt's Sample Menu: 20/80

1 glass of water once you are awake

Breakfast:
½ to 1 glass of water
1 fresh apple with skin or 1 portion of carrot sticks (eat fresh)
Your regular breakfast order
½ to 1 glass of water

Between Meals: 1 glass of water

Lunch:
1 glass of water
1 fresh orange (eat fresh, juice, or squeeze)
Your regular lunch order
1 glass of water

Between Meals: 1 glass of water

Dinner:
½ to 1 glass of water
1 portion of fresh, steamed, or stir-fried broccoli
Your regular dinner order
½ to 1 glass of water

1 glass of water 2 hours before you sleep

Sleep at least 8 hours per night whenever possible!

Purple Belt's Sample Menu: 40/60

1 glass of water once you are awake

Breakfast:
½ to 1 glass of water
1 fresh apple with skin or 1 banana
½ to 1 portion of fresh grape tomatoes
Your regular breakfast order
½ to 1 glass of water

Between Meals: 1 glass of water

Lunch:
1 glass of water
1 portion of fresh strawberries or pineapple
½ to 1 portion of asparagus (baked or stir-fried)
Your regular lunch order
1 glass of water

Between Meals: 1 glass of water

Dinner:
½ to 1 glass of water
1 portion of fresh papaya or 1 fresh pear with skin
½ to 1 portion of beans or peas (baked or boiled)
Your regular dinner order
½ to 1 glass of water

1 glass of water 2 hours before you sleep

Sleep at least 8 hours per night whenever possible!

Red Belt's Sample Menu: 60/40

1 glass of water once you are awake

Breakfast:
½ to 1 glass of water
1 fresh pear or apple with skin (eat fresh, blend, or juice)
1 portion of fresh grapes tomato (eat fresh or juice it with apple)
1 portion of fresh celery sticks (eat fresh or juice it with apple)
2 portions of 100% whole grain sandwich, whole grain cereal with almond milk, or oatmeal
½ to 1 glass of water

Between Meals: 1 glass of water

Lunch:
1 glass of water
1 portion of honeydew
1 to 2 portions of fresh salad or steamed sweet potato
Your regular lunch order
1 glass of water

Between Meals: 1 glass of water

Dinner:
½ to 1 glass of water
1 portion of fresh figs or kiwi
1 to 2 portions of spinach, lettuce, or artichokes (stir-fried)
2 portions of 100% whole grain food (pasta, bread, or rice)
½ portion of stir-fried (fish or lean meat) dish, if needed
½ to 1 glass of water

1 glass of water 2 hours before you sleep

Sleep at least 8 hours per night whenever possible!

Black Belt's Sample Menu: 80/20

1 glass of water once you are awake

Breakfast:
½ to 1 glass of water
1 fresh apple with skin
1 fresh orange (eat fresh, juice, or squeeze)
1 portion of fresh grape tomatoes or carrots (eat fresh or juice it with apple and pear)
2 portions of 100% whole grain sandwich, whole grain cereal with almond milk, or oatmeal
½ to 1 glass of water

Between Meals: 1 glass of water

Lunch:
1 glass of water
1 banana
1 portion of steamed green beans
1 portion of stir-fried spinach
2 portions of 100% whole grain food (pasta, bread, or rice)
½ portion of grilled (fish or lean meat) dish, if needed
1 glass of water

Between Meals: 1 glass of water

Dinner:
½ to 1 glass of water
1 portion of fresh berries or cherries
1 portion of fresh watermelon
1 portion of steamed brussels sprouts or baked sweet potato
2 portions of 100% whole grain food (pasta, bread, or rice)
½ portion of stir-fried (fish or lean meat) dish, if needed
½ to 1 glass of water

1 glass of water 2 hours before you sleep

Sleep at least 8 hours per night whenever possible!

17
In Conclusion

Success in life is all up to you. You and only you can change the way you look and feel. If you tell yourself that you are addicted to sugar, salt, MSG, or other unhealthy foods, you are. If you tell yourself that you truly desire better health, you can make it happen.

With this book in hand, you have the choice to be in total control of your thoughts and your health. Decide what you want and stick to it until you see the results. Your sky will clear; it is just a matter of time. Be patient, be persistent, and your life and health will change for the better.

MIND YOUR OWN WELLNESS is not about asking you to stop eating your favorite unhealthy food. Its goal is to give you a deeper understanding about what could be the causes of your overeating or poor eating habits. In addition, "The 14 Common Things To Minimize" keeps you aware of certain types of foods that could potentially bring harm to your life or the lives of your loved ones for whom you are cooking or preparing them for.

Knowing the potential risks of some foods, preservatives, and additives that you use regularly can help you and your loved ones live a healthier life. Or, at the very least, the knowledge can help you to see the connection between what and how you have eaten in the past, and you are who you are now.

Using Your Power of Thought:

Listen to your Inner Healthy Voice 80% of the time and let your Inner Junky Voice out only 20% of the time and you will begin to see positive effects in your life – *physically and emotionally*. Best wishes to you and your loved ones!

Now that you have all the 5 Color Belts' Success Formulas to help you stay on track and you have come to know your Twin Inner Voices (Inner Healthy Voice and Inner Junky Voice), the rest will all begin with just one action: Put less unhealthy food into your mouth. Enjoy the process and you will start to appreciate your body more and more, each and every day. BEST WISHES!

Please write us your success story and if possible, include your before and after pictures to:

Success@MindYourOwnWellness.com.

Share Your Success With Others!

Fresh Fruits Choices: Choose Organic if possible or available!

APPLES:
1. Fuji
2. Gala
3. Golden or yellow
4. Granny Smith or green
5. McIntosh
6. Red delicious

APRICOTS

BANANAS:
1. Baby
2. Red
3. Yellow

BERRIES:
1. Blackberries
2. Blueberries
3. Raspberries
4. Strawberries

CHERRIES

CITRUS FRUITS:

Orange:
1. Blood orange
2. Navel orange
3. Valencia orange

Grapefruits:
1. Pink
2. White
3. Pomelo (Large)

Tangerine:
1. Clementine
2. Kumquat (Sweet tart – size of a thumb – eat with skin)
3. Mandarin orange
4. Tangelo

Ugly fruit

FIGS

GRAPES:
1. Concord
2. Green
3. Mini
4. Red
5. Black

KIWI

MANGOS

MELONS:
1. Cantaloupe
2. Casaba
3. Honeydew
4. Mini watermelon
5. Watermelon - yellow
6. Watermelon – Red

NECTARINES

PAPAYAS:
1. Hawaiian
2. Mexican

PASSION FRUITS

PEACHES:
1. Donut
2. Regular
3. White

PEARS:
1. Anjou
2. Asian
3. Bartlett
4. Bosc
5. Red
6. Yali

PERSIMMONS (FUYU)

PINEAPPLES

PLUMS
1. Golden or yellow
2. Red
3. Pluots (part plum and part apricot)
4. Prune

POMEGRANATES

STAR FRUITS

Fresh Vegetables Choices:

BELL PEPPER:
1. Green
2. Orange
3. Red
4. Yellow

CARROT:
1. Baby
2. Regular

CELERY

CUCUMBER:
1. Armenian
2. Japanese

3. Mediterranean
4. Regular
5. Seedless

TOMATO:
1. Cherry (Small)
2. Grape (Small)
3. Pear (Small)
4. Plum
5. Regular
6. Vine

RADISH

Other Produce, Grains, Legumes, Nuts, and Seeds Choices:

ARTICHOKES

ASPARAGUS

BEETS

CABBAGE:
1. Bok choy (Chinese cabbage)
2. Broccoli
3. Brussels sprouts
4. Cauliflower
5. Collards
6. Gai choy (Chinese mustard cabbage)
7. Gai lan (Chinese broccoli)
8. Green or White
9. Kale
10. Napa
11. Red or Purple

EGGPLANT:
1. American
2. Chinese
3. Filipino
4. Hawaiian
5. Indian
6. Italian
7. Japanese
8. Rosa Bianca
9. Thai

JICAMA

LETTUCE:
1. Boston
2. Green-leaf
3. Iceberg
4. Limestone
5. Red-leaf
6. Romaine

MUSHROOMS:
1. Enoki (Mini or golden needle)
2. Eryngii (King oyster)
3. Italian
4. Oyster
5. Portobello (Giant)
6. Shiitake
7. White

POTATO:
1. Fingerling (Mini)
2. Red
3. Russet or Idaho
4. White
5. Yellow finn

ROOTS:
1. Beets
2. Black radish
3. Carrot
4. Daikon (White carrot)
5. Lotus root

SPINACH

SQUASH:
1. Bitter melon
2. Butternut
3. Chinese okra
4. Fuzzy melon
5. Indian bitter melon
6. Opo
7. Pumpkin
8. Turkish
9. Winter melon
10. Zucchini

WATERCRESS

Allium Family:
1. Pearl onions (Small)
2. Red onions
3. Sweet onions
4. White onions
5. Yellow onions
6. Chives
7. Garlic
8. Green onions
9. Leeks
10. Shallots

GINGER

Grains:
1. Barley
2. Brown rice or Whole grain rice
3. Oat
4. Whole wheat flour

Legumes:
1. Black-eyed pea
2. Chickpea
3. Green pea
4. Yellow pea
5. Black bean
6. Great northern bean
7. Green bean
8. Kidney bean
9. Lentil
10. Lima bean
11. Navy bean
12. Pinto bean
13. Red bean
14. Soy bean
15. White bean

Shelled Nuts and Seeds:
1. Almond
2. Flax seed
3. Pecan
4. Sesame
5. Sunflower seed
6. Walnut

Recommended Books & DVDs:

- *The China Study* by T. Colin Campbell, Ph.D. and Thomas M. Campbell II
- *Battling The MSG Myth:* A Survival Guide and Cookbook by Deborah L. Anglesey
- *Food For Life:* How the New Four Food Groups Can Save Your Life by Dr. Neal Barnard
- *Power Sleep* by Dr. James B. Maas with Megan L. Wherry, David J. Axelrod, Barbara R. Hogan and Jennifer Bloomin
- *Apple Cider Vinegar:* Miracle Health System by Paul Bragg, N.D., Ph.D. & Patricia Bragg, N.D., Ph.D.
- *Food Additives* by Christine H. Farlow, D.C.
- *You On A Diet* by Dr. Michael Roizen and Dr. Mehmet Oz
- *Everyday Cooking With Dr. Dean Ornish*
- *Fit For Life* by Harvey and Marilyn Diamond
- *Don't Drink Your Milk!* by Dr. Frank A. Oski
- *Excitotoxins:* The Taste That Kills by Dr. Russell L. Blaylock
- *Food, Inc.* by Eric Schlosser and Robert Kenner
- *The Living Foods Lifestyle* by Brenda Cobb
- *The Pursuit of Life* by Chiu-Nan Lai, Ph.D.
- *Milk – The Deadly Poison* by Robert Cohen
- *Healing Cancer & Eating* by Mike Anderson
- *The Beautiful Truth* starring Garrett and Steve Kroschel and Charlotte Gerson
- *The Great American Detox Diet* by Alex Jamieson

For more recommendations, please visit:
http://www.mindyourownwellness.com/CurrentStore.html

Recommended Books & CDs:

- *Think And Grow Rich* by Napoleon Hill
- *Believe And Achieve* by W. Clement Stone
- *Flight Plan* by Brian Tracy
- *The Missing Secret* by Dr. Joe Vitale
- *Personal Power II* (CDs) by Anthony Robbins
- *How To Raise Happy, Healthy Self-Confident Children* by Brian Tracy and Bettie B. Youngs
- *Men Are from Mars, Women Are from Venus* by John Gray, Ph.D.
- *The Gerson Therapy* by Charlotte Gerson
- *Take Control of Your Health* by Dr. Joe Mercola
- *Food Rules* by Michael Pollen
- *Try It On Everything* by Nick and Jessica Ortner
- *Move On...Your L.I.F.E. Is Waiting* by Johnny Campbell
- *Cash In A Flash* by Mark V. Hansen and Bob Allen
- *Three Feet From Gold* by Sharon L. Lechter, Greg S. Reid with The Napoleon Hill Foundation
- *The Success Principles* by Jack Canfield
- *How Would Love Response?* by Kurek Ashley
- *Your Destiny Switch* by Peggy McColl
- *Time Traps* by Todd Duncan
- *Happy For No Reason* by Marci Shimoff
- *The Psychology Of Winning* by Dr. Denis Waitley
- *See You At The Top* by Zig Ziglar

For more recommendations, please visit:
http://www.mindyourownwellness.com/CurrentStore.html

Indexes:

FREE BONUS GIFT

As a purchaser of **MIND YOUR OWN WELLNESS**, you are entitled to a special bonus from author Alex Ong.

Free subscription to **MIND YOUR OWN WELLNESS** updates. The FREE updates are as follows:

- New helpful tips!
- New contents!
- New information on other food ingredients!

To Receive Your Free Bonus Gift,

Go Here Now:

www.MindYourOwnWellness.com

click on: Free Gift

Quick Order Form

Email orders: orders@MindYourOwnWellness.com
Postal orders: OCL Publishing, Inc. Alex Ong, P.O. Box 5618, Villa Park, IL 60181. USA. **(Personal check or Money orders)**

How many books would you like to order: _____

Please send more information on:
- ❑ Speaking/ Seminars
- ❑ Mailing lists
- ❑ Consulting

First Name: _____
Last name: _____
Address: _____
City:_____ State:_____Zip: _____
Telephone: _____
Email: _____

Sales tax: Please add **7.75%** for products shipped to Illinois addresses.

Shipping by air: US: $4 for the 1st book and $2 for each additional book.
International shipping: $9 for the 1st book and $5 for additional book (estimate).

Payment:
- ❑ Check
- ❑ Money order

Credit card:
- ❑ Visa
- ❑ MasterCard
- ❑ Discover

Card number: _____
Name on card:_____
Expiration date: _____/ _____

www.MindYourOwnWellness.com

Quick Order Form

Email orders: orders@MindYourOwnWellness.com
Postal orders: OCL Publishing, Inc. Alex Ong, P.O. Box 5618, Villa Park, IL 60181. USA. **(Personal check or Money orders)**

How many books would you like to order: _____

Please send more information on:
- ❏ Speaking/ Seminars
- ❏ Mailing lists
- ❏ Consulting

First Name: _____
Last name: _____
Address: _____
City:_____ State:_____Zip: _____
Telephone: _____
Email: _____

Sales tax: Please add **7.75%** for products shipped to Illinois addresses.

Shipping by air: US: $4 for the 1st book and $2 for each additional book.
International shipping: $9 for the 1st book and $5 for additional book (estimate).

Payment:
- ❏ Check
- ❏ Money order

Credit card:
- ❏ Visa
- ❏ MasterCard
- ❏ Discover

Card number: _____
Name on card:_____
Expiration date: _____/ _____

www.MindYourOwnWellness.com

About The Author:

Beginning at age six, 'Fatty Boy' was my nickname. As I grew older, my nickname was changed to Fatty. How fun was it to be called a Fatty? I didn't care much, but I do not recall loving it. Although I was very cheerful by nature, consciously and subconsciously, I hated being fat, especially when it came to changing my clothes. I always wondered how others could stay healthy and looked so neat in their clothes and I always looked so sloppy in whatever I wore.

Years went by and not knowing what to do, I continued to eat what I wanted, whenever I wanted, and as much as I wanted. It was during my teenage years that my nickname was changed from Fatty Boy to Fatty, because I was no longer a small boy. Unfortunately, my Fatty nickname did not go away for many more years. Not even when I was in the swim team, badminton team, martial arts, and in the Army (Combat Unit) – my nickname Fatty was there to stay. Even though the Army's training was tough, somehow, I managed to eat enough junk food to keep up with my nickname Fatty.

I continued to gain weight as I grew older, because I never stopped or cut down on the junk food that I loved to eat. I loved ice cream, chocolate, chocolate milk, chips, fries, cheese, deep-fried foods, and almost everything that was very salty, sweet, or DEEP FRIED; fresh fruits and any kind of vegetables were a No-No for me then.

At age of 20 to 25, something started to change. My energy and concentration levels continued to drop. I was not able to sit through a 45-minute lecture without dozing off several times per class. My stiff neck went from bad to worse as time went by.

1st Turning Point: Meeting With My Future Mother-In-Law

At age 25, my stiff neck was hurting me so badly that I could not sit still without having to rotate my neck frequently to ease my pains. Fortunately, I continued to be myself even when I was in front of my future mother-in-law, I ate like a pig. I would eat all the things that tasted best but were bad for my health.

Then my future mother-in-law order came into play. "You have to go for a blood test," she said. What should I do? Follow her order of course – or I was probably going to lose my chance of marrying her daughter. And it turned out to be a blessing, I found out that my cholesterol was 288 at the age of 25 (a safer cholesterol zone should be less than 200, to reduce the chance of health or heart diseases). In addition, my good cholesterol (HDL) was way too low and my bad cholesterol (LDL) was way too high. What's next?

I started getting into various diet programs and went on all kinds of strict diets. Every program that I tried didn't seem to work; the weight that I lost would come back again soon after the diet program was done. One disappointment after another — but I just would not give up because I was determined to stay healthy for my future wife and my future kids. Through trial and error, at the fourth year of trying, the Color Belts' Success Formulas started to take shape. Since then, my cholesterol level and weight have been back to normal and my neck pains are gone - for years, naturally. And of course, my nickname Fatty was gone with the fat!

2nd Turning Point: A Phone Call That Changed My Life

Three days prior to September 1st of 2006, a very lovely and giving man was just chatting with me over the phone thousands of miles away. Everything seemed to be normal, as usual. This man also happened to be the man who did not give up hope on me because of my study challenged background.

Fortunately, he believed in me and gave me an opportunity to pursue my studies in the United States. It was at Oklahoma State University that I met my then future wife, Linnawaty, who later turned me into someone who loved to study, read, and write.

Sadly, on September 1st of 2006, I received a phone call from my brother-in-law in Singapore and it was about the very lovely and giving man. I lost him to a sudden massive heart attack. This man is my dear Father Ong Choon Lee.

It was the extreme pain of not having him for an extra day that inspired me to convert my years of yo-yo dieting notes into Mind Your Own Wellness to help others live their healthiest and best, not only for themselves, but also, for their loved ones too!

I sincerely hope that this book will inspire you to live your healthiest and best for yourself and your loved ones.

Background:

Alex Ong is a keynote speaker, coach, and natural health author. He is a specialist on the subjects of Stress, Healthcare Cost Reduction, Weight-Loss, Obesity, Productivity, Natural Health and Wellness - How to Reduce Stress & Weight Naturally?

His #1 mission when presenting is to provide audiences with fun and straightforward steps to improve health, reduce stress and weight naturally. What makes Alex Ong's presentation unique is, he walks his talk. He has been called Fatty Boy by others for years and he certainly know what it takes to be heavy and most importantly, he knows how to use the fun and straightforward steps to become healthy again.

Alex has been featured on various radio stations across the U.S. and internationally. He was also a featured speaker at the National Health Freedom Expo, B.I.G. National Training Conference, and Autism One Conference. He has spoken to thousands and his audience includes members of the National Institute of Health, Northwestern University, FDIC, FBI, HUD, Northern Trust Bank, National Science Foundation, US Army, US Navy, USDA, Chicago Housing Authority, Centers for Disease Control and Prevention, NASA, Holistic Moms Network, National Library of Medicine, and many more.

He attended Oklahoma State University and the University of Central Oklahoma. He holds a Master's Degree in Marketing including the in-depth understanding of Advertising, Research, and Consumer Behavior - Consumer Psychology and Buying Behavior.

In 1989, he received the Distinction Awards in Life-Saving and he was a Certified Combat Medic in the Army Infantry Unit in the 1990s. He has been in the field of sales and customer relations for over 15 years. Prior to developing MIND YOUR OWN WELLNESS's Success Formulas, he spent half a decade of his efforts as the head of the Advertising and Marketing departments in the food industry. He lives in Illinois, with his wife Linnawaty and his two children, William and Wilton.

Notes

1 Campbell T.C., and Campbell II T.M. *The China Study*. Dallas, TX: Benbella Books, Inc., 2006; 346-347.

2 *www.csun.edu/science/health/docs/tv&health.html*

3 Campbell T.C., and Campbell II T.M. *The China Study*. Dallas, TX: Benbella Books, Inc., 2006; 348-349.

4 Barnard N, *Food For Life*. New York, NY: Crown Publishers, Inc. 1993; 152.

5 *www.pcrm.org*

6 Source: J.A.T. Pennington, Bowes and Church's Food Values of Portions Commonly Used (New York: Harper and Row, 1989)

7 Barnard, N, *Food For Life*. New York, NY: Crown Publishers, Inc., 1993; 89.

8 Barnard, N, *Food For Life*. New York, NY: Crown Publishers, Inc., 1993; 89.

9 Poneman D.H, and Greene, E.A. *What, No Meat?* Toronto, Canada: ECW Press, 2003; 193-194.

10 Campbell T.C, and Campbell II T.M. *The China Study*. Dallas, TX: Benbella Books, Inc., 2006; 6-7.

11 Campbell T.C, and Campbell II T.M. *The China Study*. Dallas, TX: Benbella Books, Inc., 2006; 15.

12 Barnard N, *Food For Life*. New York, NY: Crown Publishers, Inc., 1993; 37.

13 Gittleman A.L., *Get The Salt Out*. New York, NY: Crown Publishers, Inc., 1996; 51.

14 Anglesey D., *Battling the "MSG Myth" – A Survival Guide and Cookbook*. Kennewick, WA: Front Pouch Productions, 1997; 20.

15 Michael F. Roizen and Mehmet C. Oz, *You On A Diet*. New York, NY: Simon and Schuster, Inc., 2006; 58.

16 Campbell T.C., and Campbell II T.M. *The China Study*. Dallas, TX: Benbella Books, Inc., 2006; 347.

17 Campbell T.C., and Campbell II T.M. *The China Study*. Dallas, TX: Benbella Books, Inc., 2006; 45.

18 Campbell T.C., and Campbell II T.M. *The China Study*. Dallas, TX: Benbella Books, Inc., 2006; 45.

19 Farlow C. H. *Food Additives: A Shopper's Guide To What's Safe and What's Not*. Escondido, CA: KISS For Health Publishing, 2004; 24.

20 Farlow C. H. *Food Additives: A Shopper's Guide To What's Safe and What's Not*. Escondido, CA: KISS For Health Publishing, 2004; 22, 38.

21 Statham B., *What's In Your Food?* Philadelphia, PA, Running Press Book Publishers, 2007; (1-11) 18-19.

22 Farlow C. H., *Food Additives: A Shopper's Guide To What's Safe and What's Not*, Escondido, CA, Kiss For Health Publishing, 2004; (12-15) 22.

23 Anglesey D., *Battling the "MSG Myth" – A Survival Guide and Cookbook*. Kennewick, WA: Front Pouch Productions, 1997; 50.

24 Anglesey D., *Battling the "MSG Myth" – A Survival Guide and Cookbook*. Kennewick, WA: Front Pouch Productions, 1997; 50-51.

25 *www.epa.gov; www.wri.org*

26 *www.foodnews.org*

27 Stone W. C., *Believe and Achieve*, Wise, VA, The Napoleon Hill Foundation, 2002, 39.

28 Hill N., *Think and Grow Rich: The 21st Century Edition (9 CDs)*, Wise, VA, The Napoleon Hill Foundation, 2005.

29 Bragg P. C. and Bragg P., *Bragg The Miracle of Fasting*, Santa Barbara, CA, Health Science, 238.

30 *www.cancerproject.com*

31 Maas J. B., Wherry M. L., Axelrod D. J., Hogan B. R., and Blumin J. A., *Power Sleep*, New York, NY, Quill, 2001; 6-7.

32 *www.drowsydriving.org*

33 *www.drowsydriving.org*

34 Maas J. B., Wherry M. L., Axelrod D. J., Hogan B. R., and Blumin J. A., *Power Sleep*, New York, NY, Quill, 2001; 10-11.

35 Maas J. B., Wherry M. L., Axelrod D. J., Hogan B. R., and Blumin J. A., *Power Sleep*, New York, NY, Quill, 2001; 10-11.

89324914R00112

Made in the USA
Lexington, KY
26 May 2018